NURSING LITERATURE REVIEWS

Literature reviews are undertaken by students, researchers, clinicians and educationalists – that is, almost all nurses.

Despite much excellent work, exploring the assumptions and practices that constitute searching for and reviewing literature has merit, and prompting those who undertake these activities to think critically about what it is that they are doing should be encouraged. Widely adopted approaches to structuring reviews (the "standard model") can detrimentally limit the scope or range of literature that is accessed and appraised. It is further proposed that a lack of professional ambition or confidence invests aspects of the way some nurses engage with the sources that are available to them. Across the book, parochialism is challenged. The crucial roles that values and judgement play in reviews are highlighted. It is argued that humanities and arts texts deserve, potentially, a bigger or more assured place in reviews undertaken by nurses. Difficulties in appraising quantitative and qualitative research reports are identified, and benefits linked with taking a contemplative line through the review process are considered.

This book contributes to debates around evidence-based practice and literature reviews more generally. It will appeal to anyone with an interest in professional issues, research, and the philosophy and sociology of nursing.

Martin Lipscomb is a Senior Lecturer in the Institute of Health and Society, University of Worcester, UK.

NURSING LITERATURE REVIEWS

A Reflection

Martin Lipscomb

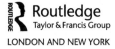

LONDON AND NEW YORK

First published 2020
by Routledge
2 Park Square, Milton Park, Abingdon, Oxon OX14 4RN

and by Routledge
52 Vanderbilt Avenue, New York, NY 10017

Routledge is an imprint of the Taylor & Francis Group, an informa business

British Library Cataloguing in Publication Data
A catalogue record for this book is available from the British Library

Library of Congress Cataloging-in-Publication Data
A catalog record has been requested for this book

ISBN: 978-0-415-79270-7 (hbk)
ISBN: 978-0-415-79271-4 (pbk)
ISBN: 978-1-315-21144-2 (ebk)

Typeset in Bembo
by Taylor & Francis Books

For Kath, Harry and Ella – still the nicest people.

CONTENTS

IN FIRST PERSON – A PREFACE

Location and appraisal can be and often are done well. Indeed, it would be presumptuous in the extreme to suggest otherwise. Nonetheless, despite much excellent work, exploring the assumptions and practices that constitute searching for and reviewing literature has value, and prompting those who undertake these activities to think critically about what it is that they are doing should be encouraged.

Reflection might suggest that, somewhat implausibly, existing ways of working cannot be enhanced. Alternatively, should it transpire that improvement is possible, it may be feasible to identify what requires attention even if the means of achieving advancement remain less certain. In either event, considering how nurses go about location and appraisal will bolster confidence and/or point towards where more productive search and review strategies can be pursued. This latter option holds out the promise of deepening understanding, and when practitioners scrutinise their activities in an informed and thoughtful manner, better nursing might result.

Positively, intelligent and challenging commentaries on location and appraisal are being developed, and a great deal of interesting discussion is taking place (see e.g. Boell and Cezec-Kecmanovic, 2011; Schryen, Wagner and Benlian, 2015; Greenhalgh, 2016; Herman, 2016; Ayala, 2018; Greenhalgh, Thorne and Malterud, 2018; Thorne, 2018b; 2019). However, problematically, outside dedicated or specialist communities, innovative work of this sort remains largely overlooked by the majority of those who perform reviews. Bothersome complications are known to exist. Yet snags are generally ignored, and nurse searches and reviews can be thought about and performed in comparatively unsophisticated ways.

Lacklustre interest in the difficulties surrounding location and appraisal may result from, in part, the ubiquity or commonplace nature of these occurrences. Thus, arguably, routinisation contributes to the perception that few substantive problems accompany enactment. And while those grappling with the processes involved can exhibit a prickly cantankerousness, excepting the annoyances and frustrations that attend performance, location and appraisal rarely excite wider passion. This is unfortunate for, inevitably, the quality (or absence thereof) of nurse searches and reviews inform what is known or not known (comprehended and believed), and this in turn impacts on how we undertake research and care for patients.

Literature reviews and nursing

To encourage the reflection that this book suggests is necessary, it is proposed that nurses need to read more deeply and widely when conducting literature searches and reviews than is currently often the case. Further, as Francis Bacon noted in the *Essays*, we should read "not to contradict and confute; nor to believe and take for granted; nor to find talk and discourse; but to weigh and consider" (1999 [1597–1620], p.114). Bacon's (ibid) statement can be understood in several ways. However, one interpretation is that, while reading can occasionally enable us to confirm or deny some contention about the world, it often proves to be of greatest benefit when, rather than concluding matters or providing amusement, reading informs thoughtful contemplation.

These anodyne assertions do not present a particularly electrifying manifesto. They are unlikely to rankle. Nonetheless, both injunctions underpin a critique of aspects of present practice and, in addition, each claim rests on premises and has implications which, if taken seriously, challenge and threaten to unravel the entrenched notions that some practitioners have about what nursing is or should be. Thus, it is argued that the manner in which reviews are conceptualised and enacted directly bears upon and is influenced by the ideas nurses have of themselves and their profession. This theme is developed across subsequent chapters. However, to indicate where discussion is heading, three sticky issues confronted by nurses involved in location and appraisal are here recognised.

First, while methodologists rightly give substantial weight and credence to science and scientific texts, that is, research and its products are described and methods for marshalling and evaluating these sources are proposed – nurses are interested in and ask questions about topics that possess scientific *and* non-scientific literatures. This binary opposition, contrasting scientific against or alongside non-scientific inquiry, can of course be objected. The bifurcation is, in its formulation, self-evidently simplistic. Nevertheless, it usefully illustrates a crucial difference between subjects that can in principle be addressed using empiric methods (broadly conceived), and subjects which defy resolution using such criteria. Pressing this point, although scientific truths are fallible and contingent, scientific methods generate probabilistic results garnering, often, considerable consensus regards their plausibility and, crudely, this situation differs markedly from non-scientific or metaphysical discourse (e.g. ethical or philosophic conjecture) where in all but a few instances agreement and closure is firmly resisted.

This much is platitudinous, yet, if we allow that nurses pose questions and take up subjects that are best tackled through reading scientific and non-scientific literatures, then in addressing what is non-scientific, non-research humanities and – possibly – arts texts might and occasionally ought to be accessed.[1] At any rate this option is not excluded.

Outside of nursing the value of non-technical knowledge is recognised (see e.g. Oakeshott, 1991 [1947]). However, problematically, work of this sort sits uneasily within commonly used models of review processes. Humanity and arts literatures are unlikely to resolve questions in the way these models presume are necessary, and although humanity and arts scholarship speaks to many of the concern's nurses have, these types of texts are not action guiding in the manner that research reports supposedly are.

Methodologists give little attention to whether or how non-research sources might be interpreted by reviewers. Yet even when purely instrumental and/or scientific issues are investigated – Traynor's "technical problems" (2013, p. 88) – it is important to remember that nurses often or always intend to use the results (data or facts) obtained to inform practice.

That facts are deployed in argument to rationalise action in the world is unremarkable. However, facts only make sense within wider landscapes of interest informed understanding, and justification inescapably contains (either implicitly or explicitly) non-factual normative and evaluative components (Trusted, 1987). Once more, the disjuncture being articulated must be treated with caution. Factual and evaluative judgements/statements are often intimately entwined, and cavalier attempts to impose too severe a demarcation between facts and values should be resisted (Berlin, 1998b [1960]; 1998c [1973]). Nonetheless, nursing theorists seem reluctant to discuss the ways in which normative and evaluative considerations influence evidence identification and use, and in both instances – when questions pertaining to topics with scientific and non-scientific literatures are asked – humanity and arts scholarship should perhaps be considered by reviewers when attentive engagement with the normative and evaluative dimensions of argument and decision making is required. That is, when insight is sought, discursive interpretation and not just data is called for (Nevo and Slonim-Nevo, 2011; Boell and Cecez-Kecmanovic, 2014).

Second, regardless of whether scientific or non-scientific sources are included in a search, reviews conducted by nurses can be narrowly and inappropriately compressed. This occurs when nurses rely primarily on nursing and medical or health related sources even when 'external' material might more comprehensively or adequately meet their needs. Looking principally or even solely at nursing and allied health literatures is disobligingly constricting when alternative sources are informative and relevant. However, should non-nursing[2] material be accessed, problems of 'overload' and comprehension are encountered when literatures lying outside discipline specific knowledge are engaged. Again, review methodologists infrequently and/or inadequately discuss these issues.

Lastly, third, the assumed need of some – probably a small subset – of nurses to vigorously protect and maintain professional boundaries and, also, a more pervasive if unquantifiable diffuse reluctance to engage with the complexity of review processes (a professional lack of ambition) exacerbates all other difficulties.

The relative dearth of serious discussion around these issues in most of the texts that nurses turn to for guidance is difficult to fathom. This lacuna materially impacts on the way reviews are performed. Further, underplaying both the value of reading and the potential role of humanity and arts scholarship to productively inform thinking/contemplation suggests that key elements or aspects of nursing's scope or remit remain underdeveloped.

In this work, it is suggested that a broader range of sources should be considered by nurses conducting reviews. The book is positively intentioned. Yet the analysis offered will not appeal to everyone. To challenge complacency a deliberately vigorous tone is adopted and, in places, an unashamedly polemical stance is adopted. More concretely, it is maintained that the manner in which we orientate ourselves towards and engage with 'the literature' cannot be disassociated from ideas about evidence-based practice (henceforth EBP), and the construction of nursing's professional identity or self-image. When undertaking literature searches and reviews, and depending upon the topic or question being addressed, it is proposed that nurses ought to read non-nursing and non-research sources as well as nursing and research materials. Moreover, and again depending on context, the objective or goal of reading may need to be revisited. That is, we ask, within a professional environment must reading always have as its prime objective the resolution of questions/problems or, alternatively, might disinterested contemplation be a legitimate goal in and of itself? To unpack these ideas widely held beliefs about nursing are tested and, inevitably, this testing may appear confrontational. Thus, adjusting the form that engagement takes will necessitate some reconceptualization of our practices and imagined community and, for some, the reconceptualization of search and review processes outlined may, in its implications, be unacceptable. Therefore, although the arguments presented are not intended to offend, it is anticipated that occasionally they will. Where this is the case, or when an instinctive "that's implausible" reaction is triggered, rather than simply proclaiming "because I don't like what you say, you must be wrong" – "why is he wrong?" might instead be asked.

Reflexivity in review processes – it seems to me

> [T]he diversity of our opinions arises not from the fact that some of us are more reasonable than others, but solely that we have different ways of directing our thoughts, and do not take into account the same things.
>
> *Descartes (2006 [1637], p. 5)*

Researchers of all stripes increasingly recognise that their biographical and culturally mediated histories influence the study process and, by implication, findings. That is, for a variety of psycho-socio-cultural and other reasons, different factors are taken into account when constructing and drawing conclusions. In response, researchers (and theorists) are reflexively situating themselves within their writing, and while this positioning takes numerous forms, through processes of open disclosure it is supposed that otherwise disguised influences and prejudices can be identified (Finlay, 2002a; Canagarajah, 2005; Nelson, 2005; Berger, 2015; Kumsa et al., 2015; Nilson, 2017 – see also Ryan and Rutty, 2019).

Problematically, however, the supposed value of these origin stories and confessionals remains uncertain. For example, once a researcher has described themselves in such and such a way, or has detailed having such and such an experience or belief, it is not necessarily clear what follows. We may, for example, be told that one or more components of the revealed past, or perhaps a special class of interaction, 'feels' or is considered important. Yet at best it is usually only possible to say that some or all of the identified factors exerted an unknown degree of influence for good or ill on unspecified aspects of the research, in indefinite ways.

This is unhelpful. Moreover, post-positivist reflexive accounts are necessarily incomplete. Storytellers may seek to present themselves in a favourable light, and external observers can often offer cogent and valid insights into an individual's life and the potential impact of experience on that person's thinking/behaviour that pass unrecognised by the individual concerned. Alternative or expanded descriptions are thus always available and this undermines (it threatens to demolish) the clarificatory usefulness of 'a' proffered history. Further, if the form of open disclosure being advocated relies upon or requires that individuals introspectively access their own mental processes in a meaningful or accurate sense, then significant criticisms of this ability must be acknowledged. Psychological research has established that people cannot comprehend their thought processes in commonly understood ways and, in consequence, self-reports of such processes – particularly those dealing with 'reasons' – must be treated with extreme caution (Nisbett and Wilson, 1977; Carruthers, 2013; Mercier and Sperber, 2018; see also O'Sullivan and Schofield, 2018, regards clinical practice).

On the other hand, in relation to searches and reviews, since the personal beliefs and values of reviewers cannot easily or always be extracted from location and appraisal processes, these things clearly matter. They are suitable objects of consideration albeit that, mindful of the aforementioned debunking of inadequate or naïve theories of introspection, it is unlikely to be the case that personal beliefs-values[3] can be 'read off' in the crude manner sometimes assumed. Further, although unacknowledged and strongly determining beliefs-values may detrimentally skew research and review findings, the idea that beliefs-values are necessarily or always problematic is rejected. Here it is suggested that rather than seeking to mitigate, assuage or obliterate such influences, where subjectivity is recognised, and following a reading of de Winter (2016), it may in some instances be supposed that the epistemological integrity of searches and reviews might instead be protected and enhanced rather than degraded. Integrity or honesty in this sense bears no clear relation to the correctness of findings. Integrity references the rounded or full logic of an argument and not the objective truthfulness of what is concluded.

Thus, whereas healthcare professionals often assume "truth is unproblematic and … the right decisions will emerge once all sources of biases are defeated" (Wieringa et al., 2018, p. 931), this is or can be a false assumption. In particular, when human affairs and the interpretation of those affairs are considered, pristine or objective facts do not exist "out there" (ibid., p. 930). Truth does not lurk, it is not sequestered behind a veil of bias and, instead, it is hereafter supposed that facts, or the knowledge/understanding we seek to obtain is "not absolute but result[s] from an interest … a bias towards a certain line of questioning that cannot be eliminated" (ibid., p. 930).

Wieringa et al. (ibid.) are concerned with decision-making in clinical encounters. That is, they focus on socio-cultural interaction and the inescapable interest informed nature of that interaction. Nonetheless, their argument – which can be accepted without adopting or rejecting positions in relation to realist vs. relativist debates – is easily stretched. And, thus, insofar as personal history contributes to the formation of beliefs and values, and where beliefs and values influence location and appraisal then, like researchers and clinicians, reviewers should not, despite the qualifications and caveats noted above, ignore their individual pasts, or attempt in every instance to repudiate biases (since the interests that biases reflect in large or small measure give form and meaning to facts/findings).

Following on from this, although this book is not a research report or review, it is a personal work. The views presented and the character of their exposition overtly capitalise on my interests, background and temperament. And while I want to row back from overly grandiose claims regards reflexivity, my history – who I am – informs what is said. Thus, I entered nursing in early mid-life having previously been employed in primarily commercial positions. The imprint of this pre-nursing experience remains with me. It colours my attitude towards healthcare organisation, as well as my perception of nursing as a discipline. Post-training, I worked in a research active and self-consciously interventionist haematology-oncology unit, I was briefly a Clinical Nurse Consultant in New Zealand, a research nurse in London, and latterly a palliative care nurse in South West England. I then tumbled into teaching, and for the past decade and a half I have lectured in higher education. In this capacity, considerable periods of mainly enjoyable time have been spent introducing student nurses to research methodologies and the ideas and activities that constitute EBP.

My career also bestrides or overlaps with periods of rapid and occasionally turbulent upheaval in nursing. I witnessed both the wholesale transition of non-clinical nurse education into university settings, and the phasing out of non-graduate routes to registration (licence). These changes have proven largely beneficial. Yet reticence concerning the trajectory of travel persists within the profession. Research and informed opinion suggest that better educated nurses outperform less educated nurses in every meaningful way (Sarver, Cichra and Kline, 2015; D'Arcy, 2016; Watson, 2016; Holloway, 2017; Jones-Schenk et al., 2017;

Aiken et al., 2018; Wangensteen et al., 2018). However, depressingly ill-considered comments continue to be voiced about the value and values of graduate nurses (Rolfe, 2015; Darbyshire, 2018; Girvin, 2018), and while it is perhaps unsurprising that ill-informed 'outsiders' misrepresent nursing, resistance to what I consider to be improvement is also discernible amongst subgroups of nurses. Thus, while education is now lodged within the academy, some nurses remain stubbornly distanced from features of scholarship that, if embraced, might positively aid search and review processes.

These bold statements are developed in succeeding chapters. Yet, here, I would just add one rider. Adapting Barnett and Coate's (2005) discussion of curricula, it could be proposed that nursing evidences, in part, a form of:

> performative professionalism in which … we witness a sliding away from the possibility of professionalism that is willing to raise complex and awkward questions about its own purposes to a professionalism that is willing simply to demonstrate its capacity to fulfil efficiently and effectively a set of roles already cast for it.
>
> *(Ibid., p. 19)*

Nursing's move into the university sector occurred at a time when the institutions involved were themselves in flux. Higher education 'reforms' emphasising efficiency and effectiveness mirrored those occurring in wider society. However, as the use of scare quotes around 'reforms' suggests, changes made in the name of these objectives are not universally celebrated. Nurses differ in the views they hold about the demands placed upon them by higher education, not least because these expectations feed into older battles concerning, for example, the nature of professionalism and the practice of nursing. Thus, taken for granted ends (e.g. providing care) can and arguably have been quietly remoulded to fit in with or meet managerialist definitions of efficiency-effectiveness that, while outwardly sensible, are nonetheless problematic (Barnett and Coate, 2005; Cope, Jones and Hendricks, 2016; Harvey et al., 2017; see also Nash, 2019); and it is not illogical or foolish for nurses to reject elements of academia that instantiate managerialist and other presumptions they disagree with. Yet, as I hope to be able to show, this is not the 'stubborn distancing' referred to above.

Linked with the move into higher education, recent decades have also seen a huge expansion in nursing research. Nurses have long distinguished themselves in this field. However, a minority occupation is now a burgeoning industry and, again, we can chalk this up as a success. Patient care is improved and improving because of work undertaken by the research community, and while significant questions and difficulties exist with aspects of the production and use of nursing research (Banner, Janke and King-Shier, 2016; Paley, 2016; Rolfe, 2016a; Saunders and Vehviläinen-Julkunen, 2018), once more, there is much to applaud. That said, an unquantified but nontrivial percentage of nurses arguably maintain a peculiarly defensive posture towards research and scholarship more generally. The relationship, assuming one exists, between defensiveness and the 'distancing' noted above is complex and opaque. Nonetheless, like distancing, the defensiveness I believe I witness has a real and adverse impact on the way we go about locating and making sense of literature.

In a similar vein although EBP is, overall, remarkably successful, we should be concerned if ideas from outside of nursing – ideas that could enrich research and patient care – pass unrecognised or, more problematically, are positively rejected when they emanate from non-nursing sources that do not fit preconceived notions of what, for example, nursing science entails (see e.g.

Parse, 2016; Watson, 2018). Reticence on the part of some nurses to actively seek out non-nursing material may be associated with the idea that nurses have a "unique phenomenon of concern" (Parse et al., 2000), possess "a unique perspective" (Ringham, 2012, p. 16), or occupy an epistemologically privileged standpoint in healthcare provision (Risjord, 2010; Rose, 2017).

The word 'associated' is important in the preceding sentence. I am not asserting that those who think nurses possess a unique gaze or "angle of vision" (Thorne, 2015) vis-à-vis patient care consciously or necessarily discount non-nursing literatures. However, if this line of reasoning is granted, few additional premises are required before it can be concluded that "high quality nursing care is nursing discipline-specific and, therefore, *must* be based on nursing knowledge as formalized in nursing conceptual models and theories" (Alligood and Fawcett, 2017, p. 6 – italicisation added). The desire to create discipline specific knowledge is understandable. It might even be useful. Nonetheless, whether nursing has a "specific domain of knowledge" (Austgard, 2008, p. 314) remains disputed. A great many (dare one say alazonic?) assumptions about the distinctiveness of nursing are likely to be made by those promoting this conception, and presuming 'high quality' nursing care '*must* be based' on nursing as opposed to non-nursing knowledge can, in my opinion, promote defensive and isolationist tendencies that rest on misconceived notions of exceptionalism.

Practice is clearly being advanced, and although change proceeds harrowingly slowly, and challenging critiques of EBP exist (Rolfe, 2005; Norlyk et al., 2017; Skela-Savič, Hvalič-Touzery and Pesjak, 2017), nurses have ample reason to be proud of their achievements. Yet while there is much to be satisfied with, considerable room for augmenting what we do remains. This augmentation applies as much to location and appraisal as it does other facets of research/EBP. However, improvement may stall unless and until the blocks on change identified here, including reticence to learn from non-nursing sources, are removed. Thus, whenever and whyever it exists, failure to engage with potentially useful non-nursing sources hobbles the scope and worth of literature searches and reviews.

'A' perspective

Homilies locating authors in their work require careful appraisal for, among other dangers, they too easily assume that individuals represent or embody caricatures of the identities they align with. Conversely, my view of nursing is heavily influenced by, as noted, pre-nursing employment and, also, ongoing immersion in and reflection on the changes sketched above. These are not the only influences on my thinking. Nevertheless, filtered through and coterminous with personal psychology, these entanglements lead me to adopt a position in relation to nursing.

Specifically, the notion that nurses care in special or exclusive ways that are unavailable to non-nurses is not one I buy into. Further, I instinctively rail against most forms of identity politics, as well as what I take to be the unthinking silliness of many group claims (i.e. claims encapsulated in phrases such as 'nurses value'). By this I mean, while we must use collective or group terms such as 'nurses' if we are to be understood (these terms facilitate comprehension), it is a mistake to confuse how description occurs (the mechanics of communication) with what is being described (van Deemter, 2010). Problematically, collective descriptors may not define real entities and/or claims attaching to these descriptors can lack credibility. For example, asserting that 'nurses value' something or other implies that *all* nurses do this thing. Yet the idea that nurses uniformly share values simply by virtue of being members of a profession is, to me, implausible (see e.g. Tuckett, 2015; Day et al., 2017; Kaya et al., 2017).

Fantastic claims of this sort are untenable because nursing is not a unitary or homogenous enterprise (Leary, 2017). And while I am reluctant to define that which refuses classification – something "definitionally amorphous" (Thorne, 2018a) – nursing might usefully be thought of as a category heading which, perhaps imperiously, corrals an array of diverse and divergent forms of activity and employments together. This description deliberately accentuates variation, and with this in mind, buffeted by enabling and disabling social and cultural structures (the exigencies of history), I see 'our' interests and values as splintered and differentiated.

Nursing is many things (Stephenson, 2017), and individual nurses, in pursuit of their own goals, cluster around what might be labelled necessary and contingent positions of contradiction and complementarity across a spectrum of issues (Lipscomb, 2014a). This awkward sentence exploits social realist terminology to emphasise the possibility that, as suggested, nurses differ from each other in thought and action. If this was not the case, if nurses shared uniform interests and values, if nursing was a homogenous entity, then it would not be sensible to talk about or describe the interactions of interest groups. Yet subgroups within nursing are identifiable (e.g. the interests of clinically situated junior nurses need not be the same as senior nurses occupying management positions). And, likewise, not only might the values held by individual nurses be as heterogeneous as those of the wider society from which they are recruited, but the relationship between personal and professionally espoused values is unclear (Drayton and Weston, 2015). Is this important? I think it is.

Location and appraisal can be and are, to repeat, often done well. And my aim in this book is simply to think through – and encourage others to think through – aspects of how these activities might be improved still further. That said, 'thinking through' is not a neutral activity. It never is. There is no *punctum Archimedis* or disinterested space. Nurses approach or align themselves to their profession in some way (how can they not?), and personal beliefs and values are always 'in play' whenever nursing is discussed or considered (hence earlier discussion/reference to de Winter, 2016, and Wieringa et al., 2018). This Preface highlights my own prejudices vis-à-vis nursing. And as will become clear, my views inform arguments across the work. Specifically, while I am minded to distance myself from the strident abrasiveness of their claims, Miers (2016) and Rosser et al. (2016) identify a persistent and deep seated anti-intellectual streak in UK nursing, and Garrett (2016b; 2018) highlights kindred tensions in North America (see also, Shields et al., 2012; Aubeeluck, Stacey and Stupple, 2016). Mindful of these undercurrents, it is argued that nurses occasionally conduct location and appraisal in ways that merit Miers (2016) and Rosser et al.'s (2016) severe and disparaging epitaph. I therefore deliberately and overtly reject what, in regards to search and review processes, are strands of thought that hold academic inquiry at arm's length. Likewise, professional defensiveness (grounded in notions of exceptionalism), and a reluctance to engage with ideas emanating outside of nursing are similarly cast-off. These problematic and complex notions have been introduced as opinions and, naturally, their meaning and significance require explanation if they are to make sense and be accepted. This explanation is threaded throughout the book, and as I hope will become clear, the issues being addressed are general in scope. They are not unique to the UK.

Last words

Petrovskaya, McDonald and McIntyre (2011) recruit the concept of 'internal critique' to describe, in nurse education, an observed "mismatch between goals, or 'ideals', and existing realities" (p. 240). In a similar spirit, this book highlights disparities between what is said and what is done. Unhelpful norms and exaggerations of instrumental reasoning are identified in relation to review processes, and insofar as these normalising discourses and logics rest on conceptions of nursing more generally, professional issues are addressed.

This is not then a 'how to' guide. A rapidly increasing array of these already exist and I am not interested in producing yet another instruction manual. Instead, in discussing neglected assumptions and practices surrounding location and appraisal, a decidedly personal and no doubt idiosyncratic viewpoint is presented (to emphasise this dimension of the work, I frequently write in first person). Further, it is assumed that readers are already familiar with the basic principles involved in searching for and reviewing literature, and rather than reproducing yet another handbook, I somewhat grandly seek to challenge prevailing customs. In this endeavour it is not expected that readers will necessarily agree with every statement made, or the sentiments they express. However, if it is accepted that alternative and potentially antagonistic ways of conceptualising nursing exist, how we go about conducting literature searches and reviews becomes a matter of debate and, ultimately, reasoned choice.

To conclude, the arguments set out may be mistaken or, even when correct, they might not be successfully conveyed. Moreover, I do not claim to offer definitive conclusions and, reprehensibly, questions are raised rather than answered. Indeed, negatively, beyond charting a direction of travel, few concrete remedies for the problems identified are offered (though given that many of the questions posed defy swift resolution, this is perhaps unsurprising). And, thus, while the absence of solutions is admittedly irritating, and a scattergun rather than a sniper's rifle is often used to target the issues discussed, beneficially the work will have merit if it stimulates others to revisit these activities. This, I propose, is a valid goal. At any rate, however wobbly, incomplete and partial my analysis is, nurses have, at a minimum, more thinking to do around this subject.

Notes

1 Hereafter, the term 'humanities' references investigation into human society and culture that is critical-speculative rather than formally empiric (e.g. theoretic exposition rather than scientific study). Further, while "All writing is creative writing" (Mitchell and Clark, 2018, p. 2), in this book 'arts' designates forms of fictive expressive composition (e.g. novels) that explore ideas and/or emotion. To aid comprehensibility (readability) both descriptors are designated as scholarship. However, clearly, not every humanity and arts text merits this appellation.
2 Throughout the book, the phrase 'non-nursing' material, source or text references research and scholarship that is conducted or written by non-nurses. It is not suggested that nursing and non-nursing research and scholarship are necessarily distinguishable in any substantive sense. Similarly, the title 'Nursing Literature Reviews' refers to reviews conducted by nurses – and it is not proposed that non-nursing reviews differ in kind from those performed by nurses. There is just research and scholarship. There are just reviews. People steer and mould these activities to address the issues that interest them and the disciplines they associate with. However, research, scholarship and reviews do not become different things when undertaken by the members of different professions.
3 Here and elsewhere (albeit erratically), a hyphen is inserted between beliefs and values. This replaces 'and'. A technical term has not been introduced.

ACKNOWLEDGEMENTS

Numerous people have commented on and contributed to the arguments presented in this book. A few voices were critical, most were supportive, several were decidedly enthusiastic – and given the subject matter that's probably a reasonable balance to strike.

Special mention and thanks go to Bernie Garrett, Kath Lipscomb, John Paley, Barbara Pesut and Sally Thorne. In addition, helpful suggestions and kind words came from Peter Allmark, Robyn Bluhm, Helen Ford, Mark Johnston, Gary Rolfe, Jo Rouse, Derek Sellman, Paul Snelling, Michael Traynor, and Lynne Williams. To everyone concerned, I am profoundly grateful for your input and assistance.

Conversations with students, colleagues and researchers have also, over the last few years, informed thinking on and around the topics discussed. It is impossible to name these people individually. Nonetheless, again, thank you one and all.

In accord with the doctrine of plausible deniability, it is important to state that the opinions and ideas expressed in this work are decidedly my own. They are not to be associated with anyone identified here.

Lastly, the first few chapters were planned and drafted during time away from teaching funded by my employer, the University of Worcester (part of the SRE scheme). Thank you for this opportunity.

1

INTRODUCTORY HARRUMPHING

- Nurse reviewers often undervalue wide reading.
- The 'standard model' or approach to searching is introduced.
- It is suggested that the standard model restrains creativity.
- A plan of the book is outlined.
- Questions regarding nursing's professional identity are posed.

Rationales supporting or justifying clinical practice frequently rely on information generated by literature searches and reviews.[1] These activities also describe bedrock or fundamental components of research and scholarship (Christmals and Gross, 2017). Done well, location and appraisal identify what is known or believed, as well as what remains to be discovered. In healthcare they enable alternative treatments and interventions to be judged and compared and, further, reviews inform discussion on the nature and scope of nursing and midwifery[2] more generally (see e.g. Perry, Henderson and Grealish, 2018; Rasmussen et al., 2018). Being able to effectively search for and review literature are, it is asserted, "core" (Lipp and Fothergill, 2015) or "essential" (Moule, 2018, p. 48) nursing skills. By facilitating informed reflection and critical thinking, these activities contribute to ongoing professional development (Rowson, 2016; Welp et al., 2018), and reviews therefore sustain practice in a manner that is just as vital and integral to patient and user care[3] as the hands-on or physical skills that are traditionally more readily identifiable with nursing.

Reviews matter

Recognising their importance, this book offers a considered but nonetheless critical commentary on popular approaches to location and appraisal. That is, models and processes that are taught to and used by most nursing students, researchers, scholars, and clinicians (i.e. almost all nurses.) Much of what is done is sensible. However, several issues impinge upon and hamper reviews and these need to be addressed.

Thus, some nurses do not see the benefit of accessing and learning from the full range of knowledge and ideas that exist. Or, if this statement is too strong, they do not act as if this benefit is realised. Moreover, commonly employed search and review strategies constrict the range of sources retrieved and, hence, nurses undertaking searches are directed to look at only a subset of the material that is available to them. If nurse reviewers are sometimes reluctant to read widely, and/or when reading occurs but potentially useful sources are overlooked, it is reasonable to suppose that location and appraisal proceed sub-optimally. In such instances understanding is degraded and those we care for – the 'objects' of research and clinical practice – may be adversely impacted.

Reading

Despite their importance, literature searches and reviews are not always respected. They do not always receive the esteem they deserve. To illustrate what is meant by this, over the past few years I have taken to jotting down the peculiar things that nursing students, educators, and researchers say about these activities and, also, the uses to which literature is put. These statements can be interpreted in several ways. However, for me, they suggest that some nurses attach little significance to location, appraisal, and, worryingly, reading.

> 'What's the smallest number of papers I need to review?'
> 'How much of this paper do I need to understand?'
> 'I don't do statistics. I don't understand them. I don't read them.'
> 'We were told, only reference research.'
> 'We were told, never cite anything that's more than ten years old.'

These comments come from pre- and post-registration (licensure) students working towards first and higher degrees and, in my opinion, they disclose a peculiar and disturbing paucity of ambition. For example, the first inquiry refers to the minimally acceptable number of research papers that need to be found and assessed for an undergraduate dissertation that, at my institution, normally takes the form of a literature review (where such work is termed an Independent Study). The question points towards an intriguing problem, and it is one I return to in future chapters. Nonetheless, within the context in which the query was posed – that is, from the perspective of an instrumentally inclined student – searching for and reviewing more papers than are needed to achieve a good or even outstanding grade represents unnecessary work. Or, put another way, given advertised marking criteria, if students can receive high marks by doing a minimum, why do more? The question therefore 'makes sense'. And if an expansive review was undertaken, and if this increased the probability that inexperience might be revealed (i.e. errors made), canny students could decide to play safe by doing less.

Alternatively, it might be objected that limiting the number and range of sources accessed during the educative process is perfectly reasonable, and perhaps this comment merely signals some such constraint. The presumption here could be that learning about location and appraisal proceeds incrementally and that, at least in the foundational or initial phase, just as a child's bike has stabilisers to prevent catastrophe and tears, so students require similar protections when learning. This objection is fine, except, it is not at all clear that the implied development occurs. It would be nice if, as beginners shrug off their novice status, the need for restrictions drop away or are removed. But when is this supposed to happen? When are the upper or higher steps of a staged approach to learning to be tackled?

Note, the reproduced comment came from a third-year undergraduate completing the largest piece of academic work in her degree. If the statement captures something important about the outlook of this student towards engagement with the literature – and I believe it does – we might ask, at what point is, or should, the anticipated transformation to take place? When will this student realise that focusing on 'the smallest number' of sources can be antithetical to real or meaningful learning? In a limited number of circumstances, and depending upon the nature of particular questions, there might indeed be a 'smallest number' of papers that can be accessed. However, while I cannot quantify or corroborate the following comment, I believe the restricted approach to reading articulated by this student exists widely if not uniformly across the student body. And once qualified (licenced), should this person, or others, turn to the literature to find out about some element or aspect of patient care, their attitude towards location could presumably be the reduced one demonstrated here.

In conversation, academic colleagues suggest it is appropriate to expect wide reading from higher but not necessarily first-degree students. I disagree. It is not unreasonable to expect that all students can and should read widely when undertaking reviews – albeit that the meaning of 'widely' presumably varies with the level and purpose of study. Further, only a comparatively small fraction of nurses subject themselves to Masters and doctoral level education, and if wide reading is a good, then my colleagues' suggestion appears to authorise or sanction poor practice among the majority of nurses (i.e. all those who do not attempt higher degrees). The proposal is also intuitively suspect.

It is not obvious that Masters and doctoral candidates have more time to read than first-degree students (see Brekelmans et al., 2016, regards continuing professional development). Many nurses pursue part-time routes through continuing and higher education, and if these students are parent/carers, and/or if they are holding down demanding clinical or administrative roles (which is often the case), they may have less available time than non-parents/carers and comparatively footloose students entering university straight from school. Lecturers might hope that post-graduate students will be favourably disposed towards reading and well informed about literature searches and reviews. However, 'hope' is a fragile basis on which to plan curricula. And if students are not required to read widely in undergraduate programs, if they are not prompted to perform reviews that do more than a minimum, it is not self-evident that this disposition and skill will spring forth *sui generis* at a later date.

To further muddy the waters, because methodological enchiridia maintain a strict focus on the formulation of answerable questions (discussed shortly), and because research evidence is prized as a search object irrespective of the type of question being addressed, students and researchers might imagine that if location criteria are appropriately and tightly specified, then a manageable (i.e. small) number of papers can and perhaps should be found.[4] This way of thinking positions reading as a burdensome chore that needs to be controlled, and the idea that contemplative engagement with the literature might have value in and of itself is undermined. Inevitably, this combination of established practice and instruction runs the risk of actively discouraging the development of good practice where good practice equates with wide reading.

The student's question also has a logic for educators since, given that large numbers of lecturers supervise even larger numbers of dissertations, common expectations need to be agreed among faculty members. Yet in stating an answer (and at the time of writing, the minimum acceptable number of sources that can be reviewed in a third-year Independent

Study is four), the rationale for executing a search is subverted. Explicitly, insofar as location and appraisal occur in order that a body of knowledge, or key understandings, or new insights/learning can be recognized, then in all but exceptional circumstances it is ludicrous to imagine these objectives are realistically or substantively achieved using pre-defined quantities of papers. This is not to say that four is too small a number (*although it is*). Rather, it is proposed that stating a number is wrong in and of itself. Instead – and to prevent the tail wagging the dog – the range, type and number of materials sought and assessed in reviews should follow the question or topic being explored.

Students do not, of course, always ask these sorts of question. Some evidence mature and developed thinking. Yet minimal acceptable expectations easily morph into *de facto* norms, and experience suggests that even talented students may find themselves nudged into conforming with parochially limiting ways of working because the alternative, wide reading, is not consistently respected by educators. Indeed, academic tutors, the very people who might be expected to challenge pinched attitudes to search and review practices, can instantiate a cramped outlook towards reading:

'I tell them, go to CINAHL,[5] one or two official sites – Oh – and the Code. That's it.'
'Students don't read. They don't have time to read. You can't expect them to.'
'If students read anything, they only read to pass assignments.'
'I say, for this assignment find fifteen references. That's enough. That's what I'd do.'
'To be honest, I don't read much myself. I only look at what's required.'

These statements were voiced by nurse lecturers in university settings, and given this, and at the risk of hyperbole, the abrogation of intellectual virtue and aspiration expressed within this advice, assertion and admission is dispiriting if not shocking. Sadly, nurse researchers sometimes fare little better:

'I tend to only reference nursing research. Is that a problem?'
'Ignore complex theory and method stuff. That has nothing to do with nursing.'
'Sociology? Okay. But no one's interested in abstract ideas.'
'I have to bumph up the literature search bit. It needs more thrown in.'
'I only read what directly bears on my subject.'

Interpretation of these comments must take into account the fact that nursing is an applied discipline. It is not a traditional academic or purely intellectual subject and, thus, perhaps inevitably, practical contingency and the immediacy and urgency of demands place students, educators and researchers within contexts and under constraints that encourage an inward facing and restrained stance to engagement with the literature to be adopted. This is understandable. Nurses are busy people. Moreover, we do not know whether the above statements exemplify common or generally held thoughts and beliefs. However, when reading is done to enrich the quality of work/thinking, cursory and superficial engagement with the literature may confuse rather than help. It must therefore be wrong – it is at least problematic – when nurses deliberately seek to limit the range of sources accessed, and it is surely misguided to search only for nursing outputs when non-nursing texts offer informative and instructive viewpoints. At root, while many of our activities focus on or coalesce around 'hands on' care, theory and scholarly discourse should not be disparaged or seen as irrelevant when, if taken seriously, this type of material might complement and advance understanding about nursing's staple concerns.

Student, educator and researcher comments can also be placed within broader conversations concerning the changing nature of higher education (see e.g. Daylight, 2017). Debates of this sort tend to be doom-laden (see Preface). They accentuate deterioration and underplay the positive. Nonetheless, while we want nurses to be interested and enthused by the subjects they study and the projects they undertake, it is suggested that proliferating 'sectoral managerialism' (itself a telling phrase), increasing financial burdens (i.e. rising student debt), and reductions in the resources available to students and researchers all combine to cut away at scholarship and education's more expansive or liberatory potential (Rand, 1984b [1972]; Rolfe, 2012; Traynor, 2013; Glaser, 2015; Graeber, 2015; Paley, 2016; Darbyshire, Thompson and Watson, 2019). That is, when students and researchers operate within clipped and disabling structures, we should not be startled when real learning is marginalised. In these circumstances modules become simply hoops that must be jumped through on the race to accreditation, and research becomes formulaic, tired and uninspired. Understandably, the adoption of narrowly restricted reading strategies is explicable if regrettable in such situations.

Yet, excuses aside, given nursing's telos or purpose, where underperformance materially and negatively impacts on research, education, and by implication practice, concern with this subject is presumably mandated from the members of a profession which claims it is "other-regarding" (Sellman, 2016, p. 24). Location and appraisal are done well. Often, they are performed superbly. However, searches and reviews of questionable quality are readily sourced and – as the comments reproduced above possibly suggest – regardless of the existence of excellence, something is seriously amiss within parts of the profession. I vehemently and wholeheartedly reject the insular and blinkered attitude to location and appraisal, reading, and cross- and interdisciplinary learning that these quotations assume. It is instead contended that, regardless of the sort of question posed, nurse reviewers need to read more deeply and widely than is at present often the case. And although the connection is difficult to substantiate, I assert that links exist between comprehensive reading, our ability to contemplate and think through what it is that we do and, potentially, improved patient care. My conception of 'good' searches and reviews require that we look more critically at our own literature and, when apposite, we need to be prepared to engage with non-nursing sources, including sources located in the humanities and arts. I further propose that checks on what is achievable must be refused, and should the approach that I advocate be adopted, some reassessment of both EBP and nursing's identity or self-image will be required.

Depending on your outlook the reassessment being promoted is either sensible and mundane, or dangerously radical. The full extent and meaning of what is proposed is made clear in subsequent chapters. However, statements by Gray, Hassanien and Thompson (2017) point towards what I have in mind. Thus, they claim that many nursing researchers turn to high ranking non-nursing journals to publish their work, and they go on to ask "Can this be good for the profession? Surely the best nursing science should be published in the best nursing journals?" (ibid., p. 2034). By reply, I would say 'not always'.

If nurses want to access the most informative material, and when that material exists in the literature of other disciplines, we should want and be prepared to read outside of nursing. Likewise, in deciding where researcher outputs are to be placed, the benefits, such as they are, of publishing in 'the best nursing journals' are just one of the factors that require consideration. Indeed, if the topic or question investigated by nurse researchers is more fully addressed in non-nursing journals, or if a non-nursing journal with a high impact factor is keen to take 'our' writing (and let us assume this suggests more people will read and/or cite that work), why not publish in that journal? Nurse researchers produce ideas and findings that are of interest to others, but if we only speak to ourselves, nursing voices run the risk of going unheard in wider society. The idea that we should want to protect our profession by sequestrating 'our' publications behind or within 'our' journals is one I am deeply suspicious of. And by extension, this leads me to a view that some may feel uneasy about. Namely, I hold that nurses need to actively push against and dismantle rather than build and maintain disciplinary boundaries. As might be imagined, this perspective has far-reaching implications for the way we read and engage with literature.

The standard model

> Increasingly, young scholars are being encouraged to formulate their literature reviews into a focused and highly structured process, along the lines advocated by the Cochrane Collaboration … for which the defining feature is a predetermined searching, screening, and summarizing rubric applied to answering a narrow research question.
>
> *(Thorne, 2019, p. 4)*[6]

Hereafter the term 'standard model' designates the typical or generic process model of searching for and reviewing literature that is introduced to and adopted by students and neophyte researchers. The term stands as a shorthand description for common practice, and in one form or another this model can be read into the work of almost every methodologist nurses come into contact with. It informs under- and postgraduate (post-licensure) education. It is the 'go to' way of describing location and appraisal.

The descriptor 'standard model' is used by, among others, Pawson (2006). He deploys the phrase in relation to systematic reviews, and he contrasts his own ideas about literature location and appraisal against or in contradistinction to this model. I do the same. That is, my ideas about review practices are presented in opposition to the standard model. The danger with this approach is that more is read into the model than can realistically be sustained, and recognising this hazard, it is repeatedly emphasised that cited methodologists – people whose work embody the model – offer alternatives and caveats to the model in their writing.

Full description of the standard model occurs over the next few chapters. However, Aveyard (2018) is here used to introduce the concept. Aveyard asserts that a "good quality" (ibid., p. 3) review "is a piece of research in its own right and has a specific *method*" (p. 3 – italicisation in original). This comment references standalone and supportive reviews, both of which follow or emulate "stages of the research process" (ibid., p. 3). Specifically, they begin with the establishment of a "defined research question which is answered by searching for relevant literature, and then appraising and evaluating that literature" (ibid., p. 3). Thereafter, results and findings are presented and "recommendations for practice" (ibid. p. 4) are made. This approach is purportedly of use to students "studying at postgraduate level … [as well as those] who are new to the process of reviewing" (ibid., p. xv).

The book from which these quotations are taken is recommended to second and third year undergraduate students at the institution where I work. It is a text I am happy to use, and if students follow its advice, they should produce material that meets module and course learning outcomes (i.e. they will 'pass'). The book is also regularly cited by students taking higher degrees, and any reasonably close reading of the text should prevent naïve searches-reviews being undertaken. This work, like other of her publications, repeatedly stresses the role of judgement (e.g. ibid., p. 9), and alterative processes and ways of structuring activity are considered (e.g. ibid., p. 38). These are the caveats noted above and, therefore, none of my comments should be construed as an *ad hominem* attack. Aveyard is a nuanced and experienced methodologist. Indeed, she is often at the forefront of discussions regards improved and innovative ways of conducting reviews.

That said, the clarifying simplification required of 'how to' texts can inadvertently mislead students and early career researchers who, subject to time pressures and insecurities concerning ability, fail to notice important qualifications in what is being articulated. In these circumstances, despite ample invitation to consider alternative strategies, vulgarised versions of what is proposed may be and often are adopted. For example, the expectation that reviews be written up in a set style can lead the unwary to suppose they must also be conducted in a processual fashion. Positively, students and beginner researchers appreciate guides that ease them into what are intimidating and difficult activities. And, by providing reviewers with a brushstroke plan the standard model delivers this structure. However, while it makes sense in the final write up of a review for appraisal to precede the discussion and/or presentation of results, we should remember that in most real-world cases analysis and interpretation are inexorably elided. Thus, appraising literature, and placing that appraisal within a context are rarely unique or distinct activities. Appraisal feeds into discussion/results and, iteratively, as discussion or interpretation advances, we may return to and reappraise material read earlier, or seek out new sources to expand upon and develop topics of interest. Therefore, unfortunately, if or when guideline stages are taken to be inviolable – and I have heard lecturers talking to students in ways that suggest this thing – something has gone awry.

Aveyard (ibid.), to repeat, encourages those conducting reviews to reflect on what they are doing, and reflection might lead to a retracing of steps or, indeed, novel experimentation when necessary (see also Aveyard and Sharp, 2013, p. 93 – where creativity is valorised). Moreover, 'kicking back' against overly standardised approaches to searching is now an established if slightly sub-rosa feature of the literature. Thus, Ayala (2018), Siegfried (2018) and Thorne (2018b) all challenge aspects of what I here define as the standard model, and in what may come to be recognised as an influential contribution, Greenhalgh, Thorne and Malterud (2018) stress the value of narrative and hermeneutic reviews over unthinking adherence to Cochrane[7] style systematic search methods. Nonetheless, while the potential for conceptual and other sorts of imaginative review to meet and overcome the problems here identified is recognised; intransigence, inertia and the deadweight of established ways of thinking and acting may prove difficult to surmount. Indeed, the standard model has, I suggest, solidified into 'the way' things are done.

Problematically, like others, Aveyard (2018) repeatedly emphasises that "All literature reviews should aim to answer a specific question" (p. 18), and to enable this thing "Finding the right question is one of the most important aspects of undertaking your literature review" (p. 19). Answering questions is a perfectly legitimate objective. However, stating that 'all' reviews should do this thing is exclusionary. It banishes other conceptions of what a review might entail. Thus, since literature searches should begin with a 'defined' question that is 'answered' using located material (primarily research reports and systematic reviews of research reports), the types of questions that can be asked and the sources which are accessed in pursuit of an answer are collapsed.

One problem with literature reviews is that they can only give you the findings from what has been studied.

(Greenhalgh, 2018, p. 42)

Limiting searches to questions that have been studied using particular forms of empiric investigation is not always sensible and it is here proposed that, in some circumstances, reviewers might 'contemplatively' explore or investigate subjects without producing action guiding findings. In advance of this argument, however, and to illustrate some of the difficulties generated by use of the standard model, problems inherent in the formulaic use of predefined inclusion-exclusion criteria when searching for literature are pointed to below and explored in later chapters. In addition, while Aveyard's (2018) "reviews are research" claim is interesting, it is also troublesome. Research is undertaken to meet a variety of objectives and it takes many forms (including, potentially, that of intellectual craftsmanship – Rolfe 2016b). Yet, asserting that reviews are research reduces the meaning that is or can be attached to research.

Inclusion-exclusion criteria

In professional contexts reading aims, ultimately, at service improvement. Moreover, service improvement is seen through the lens of EBP (in the UK practitioners are required to base practice on evidence – NMC, 2018). I intend to argue that reviewers do not always need to answer questions in the manner prescribed by the standard model (and thus 'ultimately' need not reference 'immediately' or even 'imminently'). Nonetheless, putting this to one side for the moment, the standard model is – in use – associated with the following collapse in reasoning. To answer a defined question, we are told reviewers should aim to identify *all* relevant papers. The phrase *comprehensive range* then substitutes for all relevant papers. Thereafter comprehensive range is redefined as relevant *research papers* and, finally, relevance to taken to mean research reports *of a particular type*. Locating all relevant papers thus becomes the search for a limited subset of research reports (see e.g. Aveyard, Payne and Preston, 2016, p. 1).

Issues around locating 'all' or a 'comprehensive range' of sources are examined in chapters three and four. However, here, it is simply noted that excepting the luckiest, simplest, and/or most tightly constrained of reviews, a great many papers and other materials can and often will be identified by searches. Reviewers who do not wish to examine every source located therefore need to justify why some and perhaps the majority of located sources are discarded (omitted from analysis). This justification often references inclusion-exclusion criteria. Yet as Britten et al. (2017) note in relation to qualitative reviews (though the point applies widely), while exclusion may be described, it is infrequently explained.

Thus, although students and researchers might, in writing up reviews, say something like 'the search generated one hundred hits, ninety of these were removed from analysis because they did not meet inclusion criteria', meaningful clarification rarely accompanies these statements. Specifically, bar superficialities, we are not generally told which background assumptions were operative in determining inclusion-exclusion criteria. Chosen criteria are infrequently defended, and alternative but rejected options are hardly ever discussed. That is, alternative inclusion-exclusion criteria are not described, and no reason for their dismissal is given. Inclusion-exclusion criteria can therefore appear somewhat arbitrary, and attempts to understand why a subset of retrieved materials are picked for analysis can be difficult to establish.

For example, inclusion-exclusion criteria might state that papers published within set time periods were sourced. Ten or five year cut-off frames are often used for this purpose (see e.g. Clarke, Clark-Burg and Pavlos, 2018), and whatever decision is made is or can be justified by noting the need to exclude outdated sources. However, outdatedness is context and question sensitive. This problem is picked up again in chapter five. Nonetheless, texts reporting on fast moving areas of practice (e.g. cardiology) may be outdated in weeks rather than years. While in other instances (e.g. when addressing questions related to the nature of care or compassion), the thinking of long dead Greeks can be as relevant and informative as more recent sources. These statements reference self-evident truths. However, published reviews often fail to grasp this nettle and many students – including higher degree students – skirt the topic.

Search dates can also reflect psychological rather than logical assumptions. For example, while it seems natural to set search periods at ten or five-year intervals, 'naturalness' presumably reflects the fact that we count in tens rather than any more profound reason. As a child in pre-decimal Britain, I was taught about money using both imperial and metric systems. In the imperial system a pound was made up of twenty shillings, and each shilling comprised twelve pence (120 pence or 'd' to a pound). Decimalization, or the move to a metric system, occurred in the UK in 1971. However, if this had not happened UK reviewers might 'naturally' search within twelve and six rather than ten and five-year periods. That is, when inclusion-exclusion criteria define search periods or timeframes without reference to the question or topic being explored, there is no good reason to prefer ten or five to twelve, six, three or any other number of years as a suitable cut off point. Reviewers who are as familiar with the twelve as they are with the ten times multiplication table (perhaps because they use non-decimal coinage) might 'naturally' pick twelve or some other 'obvious' subset of twelve to limit their search.

Further, when rejected papers are compared alongside included papers (and this is not always possible), reviewer decision-making can appear opaque and subjective (Greenhalgh, Thorne and Malterud, 2018). Absent clarification, it is often difficult to comprehend how inclusion-exclusion criteria are being applied, and this problem is exacerbated when poorly phrased criteria are used. Thus, criteria may be worded in lax and sketchy or, alternatively, nitpickingly precise ways. Informally phrased criteria effectively allow reviewers carte blanche in decision making (anything goes), while precisely worded criteria restrict or limit the introduction of post-location bias. Mitigating bias is generally seen as a good thing (however, note comments in Preface). Nonetheless, precision may also hamper experimentation and flexibility. Furthermore, and importantly, minor variations in phrasing – possibly very minor variations – can have big impacts on what is included and excluded from searches. Yet because the reasoning behind word choices is not generally made clear, clarity is rarely achieved.

Where good process is taken to be a measure of worth (and this assumption can be disputed), then to demonstrate the value of their outputs, reviewers need to defend the decisions that lie behind the procedures they follow. That is, reviewers must guard or protect their decisions from criticism by demonstrating that those decisions rest on valid and robust grounds. The sorts of issue identified here, however, point at just some of the ways in which this does not occur. Or, rather, occurs inadequately. Reviewers often fail to provide sufficient detail or conceptual clarity and as Britten et al. (2017) note – while this infrequently happens – those undertaking literature reviews should in this and other ways more vigorously advance "beyond description and toward theory and explanation" (p. 1370). (See also Schryen, Wagner and Benlian, 2015.)

Reviews are research – research has priority

To state the obvious, since only answerable questions can be answered, those following the standard module need to ensure these are asked. This necessity nudges reviewers to focus on particular forms of scientific and/or treatment option questions.[8] That is, questions for which answering evidence may be present. This does not mean non-scientific and non-treatment option questions are ignored. Far from it. However, insofar as non-scientific inquiry and scholarship cannot be concluded in the way 'answered' might be thought to presume, the examination of these materials is compromised. Indeed, if taken seriously, the standard model problematises, for example, reviews into ethical and normative topics or, indeed, any subject falling within the non-quantitative and non-experimental branches of the humanities and arts (future chapters develop this issue further). Associating reviews with scientific questions is synonymous with tying reviews to research and, when this occurs, non-research literatures are discounted.

Further, since nursing's version of EBP originated in and remains influenced by evidence-based medicine (Rolfe, 2016a; Broom, Mahoney and Sellman, 2017; Garrett, 2018), and because reviews are often conducted under the auspices of EBP, even within the group 'research papers', the standard model's emphasis on answerable questions unavoidably privileges methodologies and methods associated with physical science and medicine. This is worth stressing.

Aveyard (2018) says that "in most instances – maybe 95 per cent of literature reviews – you will be looking for research evidence in the first instance" (p. 46). Moreover, research is "generally undertaken according to an accepted scientific method" (ibid., p. 45). The term 'empirical' often describes this method, and "Empirical research is research that is undertaken through the observation and measurement of the world around us" (ibid., p. 45). That research is sought in the first instance does not preclude other sources being accessed in the second instance. However, linking reviews with research emanating from scientific traditions that emphasise observation and measurement blocks reviewers from exploring alternative research approaches and, also, non-research sources. Some versions of what I take to be the standard model are quite blunt on this point, and commingling reviews with research and science is widely accepted.

> A literature review is a summary of the outcomes, and critical appraisal of a number of research studies on a defined topic.
>
> *(Coughlan and Cronin, 2017, p. 2)*

> [A] *literature review* is defined as an analysis of scientific materials about a specific topic that requires the reviewer to carefully read each of the studies to evaluate the study purpose, determine the appropriateness and quality of the scientific methods, examine the analysis of the questions and answers posed by the authors, summarize the findings across the studies, and write an objective synthesis of the findings.
>
> *(Garrard, 2017, pp. 4–5 – italicisation in original)*

Moreover, where reviews occur within an EBP framework or orbit, firm linkages between science and good practice are invariably advanced.

Evidence-based practice adopts a scientific rationale and involves the selection and use of interventions based on systematic empirical evidence of beneficial outcomes. EBP is then fundamentally based on empirical science and one of its most innovative features is the clear identification of what represents the best evidence to support clinical decisions. EBP is particularly effective where research has provided evidence of the quantifiable … effectiveness of specific therapeutic interventions for specific problems.

(Garrett, 2018, p. 133)

To be clear, science and its products are unambiguously necessary and important in healthcare and nursing. My argument is not anti-scientific and, indeed, I wholeheartedly and unreservedly support Garrett (2018) insofar as he believes more and better scientific under-standing would benefit nurses. Nonetheless, a problem for those following the standard model is that research into, for example, sociology, might but need not always match what, in nursing and health science, we typically take to be empiric research. That is, researchers in this and kindred disciplines may employ methodologies and methods that do not aim to produce the sorts of conclusion that – it is sometimes presumed – stand as 'answers' in or for reviews and EBP. Additionally, while those active in the humanities might employ empiric forms of inquiry, these are not the only or primary methodologies-methods used and (to repeat) when used, empiric work in the humanities can look very different from common interpretations of 'empiric' in nursing and health science where the term routinely references particular forms of quantitative investigation.

Non-experimental studies may, like scholarship, be immensely informative. These works are often worth reading. They can be relevant to whatever question or topic we are inter-ested in, and they may and frequently should influence research and practice. However, the majority of methodological texts accessed by nursing students and researchers make it very clear that experimental studies carry particular weight in EBP, and the generalisability of findings that is attributed to this material is highly prized. Good reasons underpin such claims (i.e. experimental studies can provide action guiding evidence with clear and immediate implications for patient care). Nonetheless, it is important to stay alert to assumptions that get rolled up into the word 'research'.

Nursing interests – the things that concern us – often trespass into territory associated with social science, psychology, and we might add, philosophy, ethics, aesthetics, history, law, geography, economics, and the humanities and arts more generally. That is, nurses can wish to know about aspects of their work that are best described by or through these literatures. Debates about nursing's status as "an art, science and/or social science" (Rafferty, 1995, p. 141) are not new. Yet these discussions are forgotten when, in uncritically accepting the 'reviews are research' claim, and by overly restricting the meaning that attaches to research, significant areas of investigation and scholarship are closed off.

On the other hand

It might be objected that these assertions are too harsh. They are certainly intended to dramatize the issues I think are at stake. However, contrariwise, most methodological texts (including Aveyard, 2018) make reference to, for example, both qualitative research and vague 'other' materials.[9] If non-experimental sources are warranted search objects this pushes back against the position just advanced. And, further, additional perspectives on location and appraisal exist.

Less pressure is, for example, placed on qualitative researchers to follow the standard model's format since in particular instances (e.g. grounded theory) supportive reviews are undertaken late in the research process (Barker, 2013). Moreover, a comparison of terminology presented in three of the better texts used by nursing students and researchers reveals that, although considerable overlap in nomenclatures exist, variation in search and review descriptors is apparent. The significance of this variation is open to dispute. It could point towards confusion and/or it might reference the difficulty of establishing meaningful category descriptors. Nonetheless, the possibility of alternative routes through location and appraisal is at least held open.

For example, while Booth, Papaioannou and Sutton (2012) do not specifically target nurses, their book is cited by nurses, and this work identifies twelve types of review. These are labelled critical reviews, integrative reviews, literature reviews, mapping reviews/systematic mapping, meta-analysis, mixed studies reviews/mixed methods reviews, overviews, qualitative systematic reviews/qualitative evidence synthesis, rapid reviews, scoping reviews, state of the art reviews, and systematic search and review (pp. 26–27). Alternatively, Aveyard, Payne and Preston (2016) designate six categories of review in a book aimed at postgraduate health and social care workers. These are termed systematic review with meta-analysis; systematic review with meta-aggregation; systematic review with an interpretation: meta-ethnography, thematic synthesis, meta-synthesis; systematic review of mixed methods studies with interpretation: critical interpretative synthesis, integrative reviews; systematic reviews to develop theory: realist reviews, narrative synthesis; and systematically undertaken overviews: scoping studies, bibliometric analysis (p. 17). Additionally, in a list that explicitly recognises its non-exhaustive status, Coughlin and Cronin (2017), who aim their work at nurses and health and social care workers, identify the following fifteen commonly used descriptors for types of literature review: narrative, traditional, descriptive, standard, integrative, scoping, qualitative, concept analysis, realist, rapid evidence, systematic, meta-analysis, meta-synthesis, meta-summary and meta-ethnography (p. 11).

Many other listings could be cited to evidence ways of working that extend and contradict the standard model, and if students and researchers used the leeway available to them in these works – that is – if they stepped away from an overly close association with the standard model, if they accessed a diverse range of literature sources, and if those sources were flexibly interpreted, contrasted, and combined; then the issues I here present as problematic could be dismissed. However, this rarely happens. Assumptions inherent in the standard model trickle through most nurse writing on this subject, and despite their sophistication, its limiting features emerge even in the work of those authors cited above. Further, it is debateable whether these 'better' texts give readers the detail that would be needed to, for example, perform a competent meta-ethnographic review. And, if this detail is absent, students and researchers who might be prepared to be adventurous, will find their enthusiasm thwarted (this issue is discussed further in chapter three).

Thus, despite the possibilities that exist, when we look at the sorts of journal article and book that students and early career researchers turn to, it is clear that the question-answer format dominates. Statements to the effect that: "The first step in searching for evidence … [requires that you] identify a question" (Barker, 2013, p. 59), and "The purpose of a literature review is to collect the relevant evidence to answer a clear, concise question" (Rowson, 2016, p. 93) abound. Moreover, the generality of texts doggedly require that the subjects addressed be ones that can be resolved by reference to research and, additionally, distinct biases in the type of research capable of answering questions is discernible (Rycroft-Malone et al., 2004).

In summary, a potentially helpful if simplifying guide (the standard model) has become a constraining convention. Further, while numerous alternative strategies are available, students and researchers seldom take advantage of these freedoms. That is, reviewers underplay or fail to recognise that questions do not always have to be answered by reference solely to research and recommendations for practice described. That these objectives do not need to be prioritised in every instance might seem odd. Nursing is after all a practice-based discipline. However, along with the idea that non-nursing and non-research sources be considered, this is precisely what is being argued.

The book in outline

It has been proposed that wide reading is not prized by all nurse reviewers. It was also suggested that when reviewers follow what is here defined as the standard model, a constricted range of sources and objectives are privileged.

Chapter 2 explores and further develops the concept of a standard model. The claim that nurses ask answerable and unanswerable questions is unpicked, and it is asserted that location and appraisal are inherently judgemental or interest led. The value of wide reading is again valorised, and problems associated with ignoring relevant but undervalued data and ideas are recognised. Thereafter, Chapters 3, 4 and 5 use an example 'ordinary search' to structure a series of challenges to what has become usual practice. Thus, conceptual muddle is identified, the role of values and beliefs in reviews are noted, and the possibly beneficial inclusion of non-research and non-nursing sources in searches that aim to inform practice and/or research is discussed.

Specifically, Chapter 3 alleges that basic or grounding concepts in review processes lack clarity. For example, ambiguity in the wording of review purposes and questions can be a source of confusion, and important terms such as relevance and comprehensiveness lack substantive meaning. Chapter 4 outlines a potentially positive role for non-research and non-nursing sources in reviews. The significance of reviewer judgement is emphasised, and the place of beliefs and values in evaluation are assessed. In Chapter 5, a 'new' search is conducted to illustrate deficiencies in the standard model approach. Epistemic theory (theory about knowledge) is introduced and research and non-research scholarship are contrasted. It is argued that non-nursing and non-research sources may be credible but overlooked sources.

Chapters 6 and 7 offer a change in focus. Chapter 6 looks at the way reviewers engage (or more often fail to engage) with the statistical tests that appear in quantitative papers. It is claimed that a lack of preparation (education) makes it difficult for nurses to understand how quantitative findings are derived from statistical tests in anything other than a trivial sense and this, it is stressed, matters. Significantly, if understanding how findings are derived is a necessary part of the review process – and if meaningful rather than superficial understanding is required before findings can be declared warranted or trustworthy – then it is difficult to see how or in what way findings can justifiably be accepted and/or used when the statistical tests used to identify them are not understood. It is further suggested that advances outside of nursing involving trends or developments that are often described using the label 'big data' compound the problems in comprehension that nurse reviewers face. By contrast, in Chapter 7 the disputed and awkward place of qualitative research in reviews is addressed. Problems surrounding generalisability and synthesis are outlined, and it is proposed that 'active citation' represents another possible advance in thinking that, occurring outside of nursing, nurses have yet to acknowledge.

Chapter 8 concludes the work. Here an admittedly tentative argument in favour of 'contemplative reviews' is advanced and, in this way, assumptions threaded throughout the book are tied together. Specifically, writing on the nature and value of contemplation as a good in and of itself is recruited to invert over-reliance on standard model presumptions. It is suggested that the place and role of values in reviews require considerable further methodological development, and it is proposed that the range of material that might legitimately find a place in nurse searches should be opened up.

A space between thought and action

Throughout the book, and following the lead if not the letter of Harden and Thomas (2005), and Whittemore and Knafl (2005), it is proposed that the range or scope of location and appraisal needs to expand if nursing is to engage seriously with many of the questions and topics that its members, as well as those we minister to, care about. To this end, and mindful of the work of Lacan (1998 – see also Krips 2010), it is proposed that, like other healthcare professionals; while nurses want to think about or model professional knowledge and understanding in ways which assume some sort of 'God's eye' or authoritative gaze over events is desirable and possible, this goal is frequently and disturbingly thwarted. That is, although understanding aims at grasping and ordering the key facts and pertinent features of patient problems, this objective is not always achieved. Indeed, in response to all but the simplest of treatment option questions, epistemic certitude is often unattainable. And, while professional esteem and the control of anxiety is closely tied to the assurity of knowing (Ellis, 2016), and those we care for demand the type of unfaltering competence that expertise embodies (and this is what we say we provide), mastery is seldom evidenced.

Thus, although those who search for and review literature want to comprehend what is known – what is known – even when this is apparently clear cut, may not justify confidence in action. Researchers are often acutely aware of deficiencies and gaps in the suppositions they accept, and in clinical contexts, while the literature might strongly suggest that 'this' rather than 'that' is the case, and professional expertise clearly exists, doubt ordinarily obtains. Indeed, as soon as our hard-won knowledge is deployed to inform decision making with real people in real situations, so many 'elements' or 'dynamics' must be taken into account that the only rational position to adopt is one of epistemic humility. This differs from disabling scepticism or facile ennui and, instead, it is merely recognised that while understandings built upon research evidence are fallible, contingent and provisional, and insights derived from non-research sources are perforce fragile, professional duty dictates that we continue to work modestly towards the 'best' understanding that is available to us. And, in pursuit of this goal, limiting the sources we access and engage with is self-defeating.

If nurses (students, researchers, scholars, clinicians) are to benefit from the literatures that exist, they might therefore consider three possibilities. First, we can concede that full comprehension, like total mastery, is seldom possible and more commonly we mostly only ever see 'through a glass darkly'.

Second, we should value the sort of cautious and considered reflective or discursive thinking/engagement that is, today, at odds with the hurried pace of research, education and clinical practice (Rose, 2013; Ofri, 2019). Specifically, we must question the idea that location and appraisal are – or are simply – technical activities that can be 'applied' and accomplished efficiently. Sometimes these descriptors are appropriate. However, where our aim is deep rather than superficial understanding, when we actually want to map what is known, or comprehend the key aspects of thought around a subject, then it is unlikely these activities can be rushed. They take time. Indeed, the relationship, such as it is, between learning and behaviour is often complex and extenuated, and what we take from the literature need not map onto action in any straightforward sense. A space therefore needs to be inserted between thought and action. For, as Matthew Arnold (2009 [1869]) long ago noted, the ability to critically reflect is threatened both by the urgency of immediate practical considerations, and in the face of complication, our tendency to unthinkingly place faith in established and disingenuously simplifying systems. Huxley (1937) advances remarkably similar arguments.

Third, having recognised that opacity in understanding is inevitable and that ambiguity is normal, and having surrendered the idea that nurse generated research findings are all that need be considered, we can discuss whether professional expectations and customs, actualised as the 'silos' (Tett, 2016) we operate within, block or hamper wide reading and meaningful engagement with the literature. That is, the felt need of some nurses to protect and maintain professional boundaries, and a more general lack of ambition, should be confronted and repudiated.

Reimagining professional identity

While benefits undoubtedly accompany professionalization, overemphasising nursing's uniqueness (exceptionalism) leads to the erection of barriers around our field of expertise/ operation which – wittingly or otherwise – foreclose on meaningful cross- and interdisciplinary learning. These barriers, which might be likened (somewhat dramatically) to Weber's (2012 [1905]) *'stahlhartes Gehäuse'* or 'iron cage', are unhelpful. They reinforce the idea that searches and reviews conducted by nurses should limit themselves to particular types of literature (i.e. research) and disciplines (i.e. nursing). However, if these ideas are rejected, some adjustment to nursing's professional identity and self-image will be necessary. This commits me to advancing a small 'p' political position that, as previously emphasised, some nurses may find unpalatable; and with regard to this commitment, I here consider it important that two tightly interlinked positions be vetoed.

First, I do not accept that "[i]t should be mandatory that all nursing research activity in whatever form should have meaningful links with clinical nursing and patient care" (Cowman, 2017, p. 235). Whether undertaking a supportive search as part of a research project or, alternatively, a standalone review (I interpret 'research' broadly), nursing students and researchers will generally evidence these links. But why mandate this? Students, researchers and clinicians must be allowed to engage with and in conversations about abstract and/or non-nursing (non-patient care) issues. The scope and remit of these conversations need not be prescribed. However, for example, they might involve the development, revision or consideration of conceptual, methodological and/or theoretical tools. Or, since nurses operate across health and social care – because we can be worth listening to – nurse researchers and scholars could explore and advance policy and other critiques (perhaps concerning organisation, structure, and healthcare financing) that step beyond 'meaningful links with clinical nursing and patient care'. Wide reading and close engagement with other disciplines may tip nurses away from a sole concern with hands-on care. Nonetheless, these activities and the conversations they generate have potential merit, and it seems foolish to censor or disbar them on principle. Research and scholarship can, like other hybrid roles, divert nurses from the bedside (Cooper, 2017). However, while no guarantees can be given, explorations of this sort might feed back into the development of more nuanced and sophisticated understandings of clinical practice at a later date, and if they do not always do this, we can live with that.

Second, methodologists such as Aveyard, Payne and Preston (2016), while permitting reviewers to make use of theories "relevant to your academic discipline" (p. 52), actively seek to hedge non-disciplinary encounters. For example, while psychologists are allowed to "refer to psychological theories" (ibid., p. 52), we are told this reference should not (is unlikely to) extend to "sociological theories even though some sociological theories might have clear relevance to your work" (ibid., p. 52). Aveyard, Payne and Preston offer practical guidance to reviewers. Yet many and perhaps a majority of the topics we interest ourselves in – as primary researchers and literature reviewers – are not discipline specific; and the above comments could be read as suggesting that even when it has 'clear relevance to your work', nurses should not engage with psychological or sociological or ethical or any other literature when that literature falls outside our discipline. This would be absurd. Moreover, as a simple practical matter, how, for example, unacceptable non-nursing ethical or sociological literature/theory is to be differentiated from acceptable nursing ethical or sociological writing remains unclear (Lipscomb, 2014b).

If accepted, Aveyard, Payne and Preston's (2016) claim neuters the ability of nurses to explore anything other than a small rump of discipline specific theory. Further, the outlook encapsulated or assumed by Cowman (2017) arguably problematises or undercuts important facets of meaningful interdisciplinary cooperation and learning. I do not suppose this is their intention, and Aveyard, Payne and Preston (2016) stress the role that judgement plays in determining relevance. Nonetheless, do we want to say that non-nursing theories are or cannot be legitimate sources of information or insight? Is this feasible? Should nurse educators, for example, avoid engagement with wider pedagogic literatures? Ought researchers to ignore the work of non-nursing theorists when that work might productively inform their studies? Or, are we saying clinicians are disbarred from reading government and other reports about healthcare when those sources do not speak only to patient care, and/or emanate from outside our profession?

These questions do not invoke or rest on straw man arguments. These types of question, although palpably silly, must be asked of anyone who wishes to limit reading and/or cross-disciplinary partnership.

Endnote

To develop the themes explored in this book I draw, as stated, on long experience in higher education. In this capacity, I have undertaken and participated in research, I have introduced students, researchers and clinical nurses to the joys of literature searching – and I have attempted, together with colleagues, to establish the epistemological status and use value of research reports and other documents. Throughout these endeavours I have repeatedly been struck by contradictions and anomalies between how location and appraisal are described or taught and what actually occurs or is attempted. That rhetoric and reality diverge is unsurprising in this as in other matters. Nonetheless, the significance and possible implications of this divergence remain underexplored.

Thus, in reality, finding and making sense of literature is often a headache for students. For researchers, locating and appraising previously conducted studies easily becomes a necessary but unexciting prelude to the more glamorous tasks of collecting and interpreting new data. Identifying supporting texts and background and further reading for students can degenerate into just another wearisome chore to be endured as educators hurriedly prepare teaching resources. And, for clinicians, since the exhortations of governing bodies regards keeping up to date are rarely accompanied by the provision of suitable resources that would enable this to happen (e.g. 'set aside' work based study time – Alving, Christensen and Thrysøe, 2018), it is hardly surprising that many practitioners seldom read beyond the shortest of bulleted guidelines.[10] Against this background, the arguments presented here are intended to stimulate discussion and interest into what, for many, are a decidedly arid set of activities. Negatively, critiques of the sort offered in this book can appear unrealistic, idealistic or – worse – needlessly and negatively destructive. Current methods of proceeding are believed to 'work'. Or, they are seen as satisfactory. On the other hand, if location and appraisal can be even marginally improved then, given the undeniable importance of these activities and their potential ramifications vis-à-vis practice, that possibility should be explored. Admittedly, my position presents nurses with difficult tasks. Nonetheless, ultimately, my hope is that concrete benefits, namely improvements to patient care, may accompany or follow on from discussion of these subjects.

Notes

1 Throughout the book searches and reviews are treated as alternative ways of describing the same activities. Of course, these terms can be disaggregated. They can be treated discretely. 'Searching for' may be tied to location and 'reviewing' might be associated with appraisal (i.e. evaluating or making sense of what was discovered). However, in colloquial and scholarly use these descriptors are so tightly coupled that, for all practical purposes, they are effectively synonyms.

2 Henceforth 'nursing' denotes both nursing and midwifery. I appreciate this is annoying for midwives who may understandably feel that the uniqueness of their profession is being denied. Please accept my apology. However, the alternative, forever listing 'nursing and midwifery', is somewhat clumsy.

3 Numerous terms describe those we care for – e.g. patient, user, client, partner, etc. For brevity's sake, 'patient' hereafter designates all such categories.

4 Sellman (2019) develops a not dissimilar argument – e.g. one concerned with limiting reading – in relation to required and recommended student texts.

5 Cumulative Index to Nursing and Allied Health Literature (CINAHL): "the most widely-used and respected research tools for nurses, students and allied health professionals around the globe" (EBSCO, 2018).

6 These comments reference qualitative synthesis. Moreover, Thorne (2019) does not use the term 'standard model'. Nonetheless, this is – in my view – what she describes. Alternatively, Greenhalgh (2018) cites the 'standard format' (p. 49) of teaching research appraisal skills and, again, I read this phrase as referencing (in broad terms) what I take to be the standard model.

7 The Cochrane Collaboration – https://www.cochrane.org/

8 Phrases such as 'scientific' and 'non-scientific questions' are henceforth used as shorthand ways of describing questions that can be asked of topics and/or problems for which, potentially, scientific and non-scientific literatures exist.

9 See, for example, Aveyard (2018) pages 70–71. Here it is noted that, while what is sought depends on the research/review question set, primary research reports should nonetheless be prioritised. Anecdotal and opinion papers may be sourced when research evidence is unavailable. Yet reviewers must be mindful of the 'weak' status of this material. The exception to this involves reviews dealing with theory and policy literatures. A one paragraph example pertaining to obesity and the media is provided. However, meaningful discussion on how to locate, analyse and use non-research material is not provided.

10 Obviously, clinicians read in their 'own time' (i.e. outside of work). However, given that home or personal life is often exceedingly busy, this reading may not be as extensive as ideally we should like.

2

TWO TYPES OF QUESTION

- Nurse reviewers ask questions that are answerable and unanswerable in principle using empiric or scientific methods.
- Location and appraisal are inherently judgemental in character.
- Reading widely is (again) valorised.

Students and researchers tend, regardless of academic level, to be introduced to location and appraisal *as if* these activities chiefly or even solely involve enacting a series of agreed procedures or tasks. That is, despite the availability of alternative approaches, nurses often learn about and come to conceptualise location and appraisal as a sequence of settled steps and technologies that must be mechanistically worked through. Indeed, while, as stated, skilled methodologists stress the role that judgement and creativity play in review processes, what is required may come to be envisaged as something relatively straightforward. Thus, although searches are time consuming and often exasperating, operating within the standard model, searchers are encouraged to begin by defining an answerable question. Inclusion and exclusion criteria are then set, specialist health related and professional databases and websites are interrogated using limited and limiting sets of keywords, and particular forms of evidence (principally research reports and systematic reviews of research reports) are identified. Thereafter a subset of relevant papers is selected for further review, the method and methodological robustness of located texts is assessed, and the findings of papers deemed valid and reliable are provisionally accepted as having use value for or in practice/further research.

The standard model and evidence-based practice

From the perspective of an educator, disaggregating reviews into a succession of teachable moments and gradable skills is helpful. It transforms something daunting – it converts student aporetic distress – into that which is comprehensible and 'safe'. And while the practicality of this approach may be challenged, from the standpoint of a tutee or researcher, this essentially reductive strategy is unremarkable. Thus, almost every 'how to' manual presents location and appraisal as activities that can be mastered in a stepwise fashion. Journal publication requirements normalise or reinforce these assumptions by restricting the write-up of searches in research reports to a bare synopsis of completed and apparently trouble-free (and generally theory-free) actions. Standalone reviews, both non-systematic and systematic, similarly underplay the complexity and judgements contained within the processes they describe. And the performative character of particular versions of guideline construction reproduce this methodology.

Other disciplines and professions entertain kindred ideas, and the approach to location and appraising literature outlined here is not unique to nursing (e.g. see Rosenberg, 2017). Nonetheless, these ideas receive a distinctive twist in nursing and, as noted, the power and prominence of the standard model rests or relies in part on the influence that biomedicine and the biomedical sciences exert on nurse academics, educationalists, researchers and clinicians (Playle, 1995; Lavin et al., 2002; Hudson et al., 2008; Mills and Hallinan, 2009; Baldi et al., 2014; Rosser, 2016; Mackey and Bassendowski, 2017). This influence is mostly to be welcomed and applauded. Nonetheless, it carries a downside and, problematically, while introducing students and researchers to literature search strategies that focus on the location of primary research reports and systematic reviews of those reports has huge worth, these types of source do not adequately recognise or address questions pertaining to value, meaning, or more generally, the positive if disruptive potential of critical thinking (Springer and Clinton, 2017).

Two objections might be made at this point. First, it could be argued that professional instruction should refrain from involvement in open-ended value-meaning questions and, instead, nurse education and research should embrace biomedical norms and concentrate on developing, transmitting and inculcating knowledge of human anatomy, physiology, pharmacology, disease processes, *etcetera*. That is, nurses ought to primarily focus on knowledge derived from physical and medical science, and comprehending an agreed albeit mutable corpus of 'hard' health related facts should take precedence over, for example, ethical and normative cogitation.[1]

I have some sympathy with this position since, when I am ill, I want the team caring for me to principally have knowledge of whatever ailment troubles me, and although my next comment trivialises a complex subject – while being 'nice' is important, technical competence is vital. Alternatively, even though I would welcome a greater focus being given to physical and medical science in nurse education, if we grant that nursing involves more than the application of scientifically derived knowledge, we must concede that many of the concepts which underpin its practices rest, insofar as they rest on anything, on ideas and literatures that are unconnected or only tangentially connected with those employing traditional scientific methods. Therefore, although, beneficially, evidence based medicine's preoccupation with answerable treatment option questions continues to facilitate great progress across numerous aspects of healthcare (including nursing), and it remains the case that 'we' have a great deal still to learn from this perspective (I am not and do not wish to be perceived as decrying this approach to knowledge creation/application), in addition to biomedical and traditional laboratory derived data, nursing employs and relies on alternative knowledges and ways of acting. That is, human experience cannot be fully described or explained by medical science, and to address these 'broader concerns' (i.e. broader than purely biomedical questions), nursing employs concepts and embodies practices that are associated with or emanate from what might sweepingly be called the humanities and arts (Springer and Clinton, 2017).

These assertions do not, I hasten to add, reference Ryle's (1945) distinction between 'knowing how' and 'knowing that'. Nor do they lend succour to woolly holism or the wackier hippy-dippy fringes of nursing discourse. We should have no truck with complementary nuttiness, essential oil tomfoolery, 'Unitary Caring Science' (Watson, 2018), or "mystical ... explanations of care" (Garrett, 2016a, p. 182 – see also Garrett, 2018). Further, while the standard model of reviews gives priority to a version of scientific inquiry; reviews and/or EBP do not constitute "a good example of microfascism ... in the contemporary scientific arena" (Holmes et al., 2006, p. 180). Such talk is nonsense.

Instead, the above comments simply recognise that nursing includes within its compass a variety of activities, but if biomedically derived methods of literature location and appraisal overbear, and if, in consequence, we exclude this wider reality and heritage then, insofar as they cannot accommodate themselves to the biomedical 'way', current methods of searching for and reading literature are perforce inadequate. That is, they are inadequate to the extent that non-scientific literatures are ignored. Default assumptions, imported into nursing primarily from medicine, assumptions that collapse or constrict relevance, therefore forfeit elements or dimensions of nursing that refuse such treatment, and as will be argued, this forfeiture comes at a price.

Second, it could be claimed that qualitative research already examines value and meaning questions – so what's the problem? A great deal of this material perfuses the nursing literature, and if the findings of these studies adequately address value and meaning questions then, tautologically, those questions are dealt with. The role and status of qualitative research in reviews remains, however, controversial (this is discussed in future chapters). In part, controversy mirrors the contested nature of qualitative research. However, here I simply assert that value and meaning questions are not concluded through reference to qualitative studies, and (a different point) the ability of reviewers to successfully integrate qualitative work into reviews is disputed. That value and meaning questions are not decided simply through qualitative research is an important claim, for if qualitative studies were all that was needed when addressing these questions, a key plank in the argument favouring reading non-research sources is kicked away.

"May God us keep From Single vision & Newtons sleep"

This subheading reproduces a line from William Blake's letter to Thomas Butt (Keynes, 1980 [1802]). It expresses repulsion towards the one-dimensional mind-set or 'single vision' of those who suppose Newtonian or classical science can answer all and every question. Logical limits to scientific explanation may or may not exist (Barrow, 1998; Rescher, 1999; Dupré, 2001). However, absent a crystal ball it is impossible to foretell how far science can or will proceed. What we do know is that science – for all its many and abundant blessings – cannot, at present, address the totality of the questions and topics that interest us and, therefore, if current definitions of review processes exclude or downplay the importance of non-scientific sources, then too bad for those definitions. They can be remodelled.

I intend to argue that reviews can explore as well as answer questions and, further, the questions that emerge from a review can be as important and interesting as those that are answered. Rather than accepting the standard model's precepts, let us then tweak the definition of reviews. Thus, despite the variation in types of review noted in chapter one, it might be assumed that, however they are envisioned, reviews share an essential or common purpose. Namely, while location and appraisal aim to buttress, deepen, develop and/or advance knowledge, understanding, and insight – and these might be considered diverse objectives – it could be supposed that reviews are undertaken to, put simply, learn from the literature. Negatively, this definition leaves the meaning and nature of learning indeterminate. However, no mention is made of answering questions (though this goal is not excluded), and the forms of literature needed to be sourced to facilitate learning remain open.

The benefit of describing reviews in this more expansive way becomes apparent when we recognise that nurses are engaged in broad domains of activity and endeavour (e.g. patient and family focused physical, social and emotional care/support, organisational administration and management, research, teaching, etc.), and in consequence, inquisitive nurses take interest in different types of problem. Different problems generate different questions, and while this statement is platitudinous, failure to recognise and tease apart the meaning and repercussions of differences in the questions nurses ask can throttle or misdirect location and appraisal. More precisely, acknowledging that some questions cannot be answered in the way demanded by the standard model does not mean those questions are illegitimate. And the difficulties reviewers face when confronted by the requirement that they answer questions against criteria that assume traditional scientific norms is resolved if, in some circumstances, we refuse those norms.

Answerable and unanswerable questions

While science and its products are immeasurably important in healthcare, science's reach and remit have limits. Quantitative and qualitative studies address some but not all of the questions that concern nurses – and students, researchers, scholars, and clinicians can be drawn to problems and topics that are necessarily unanswerable using scientific or objective criteria. For example, questions pertaining to normatively evaluative matters (questions of value and meaning) are rarely concluded using purely empiric data (broadly conceived). Indeed, questions exploring these topics can be and often are unanswerable in a definitive sense. Critically, the descriptor 'unanswerable' is not used here in a derogatory or pejorative fashion. It simply references the impossibility of argumentative closure in particular instances. It points at what is self-evident, namely, that people reasonably and rationally disagree on issues that cannot be resolved using scientific methods and scientifically derived data. And, often if not always, the sorts of issue addressed by these questions are fruitfully or best met using humanity and arts literatures.

Discussion could, at this point, lead off into the darker realms of philosophy of science and/ or epistemological musings. These literatures are interesting. However, here I simply want to stick with the distinction (admittedly crude) between two types of question. On the one hand nurses ask and turn to the literature with questions that are answerable in principle. By 'answerable' I mean, questions that might be concluded and an agreed or consensual answer established – albeit provisionally – for many if not all interested parties using established scientific and related forms of inquiry. We will call these answerable or scientific questions.

For example, the question: 'What is a safe dose of 'x' to administer?' is amenable to scientific investigation and potential resolution. Thus, assuming the quantity, strength, and method of administration of whatever medication is being considered is specified, and against pooled observational (quantified) data, it may be possible to accurately estimate benefits-harms against agreed health objectives/outcomes for identified patient groups. Anyone undertaking a literature review which focused on locating research might, in this instance, establish recommendations for practice detailing safe aggregate dose ranges. Treatment option questions are generally of this type.

Alternatively, and as stated, nurses also interest themselves in unanswerable questions. (The existence of which is presumed by methodologists when they state that answerable ones be chosen for review.) Unanswerable questions address topics that are not amenable to scientific resolution. Unanswerable or non-scientific questions are not in principle answerable (usually) in the manner described above. (I put to one side assuredly scientific questions that cannot, at this juncture, and perhaps for ever, be answered.) Many variants on this type of question exist and future chapters explore some of these options (e.g. questions that invoke and invite aesthetic, political, professional and socio-cultural consideration). However, as noted, ethical and moral questions provide obvious examples.

Thus, in my role as educator I have met several students who wanted to explore the subject of witnessed resuscitation in their third-year dissertations (or Independent Studies). Royal College of Nursing (2002) guidelines offer invaluable support here – and many other helpful documents exist. Nevertheless, confronted with (sometimes) confused and/or unclear 'real world' expectations, students must take a position on whether they intend to actively attempt to facilitate relatives to be present during arrests. Recognising ambiguity in practice generates concerns/anxiety and, interestingly, students consistently articulate these concerns by asking questions such as 'Should nurses facilitate witnessed resuscitation?' or, 'Should witnessed resuscitation be allowed?' Since the students who asked these questions had or would be going into the emergency department (A&E), these seem like reasonable questions to pose. That is, questions of this sort examine aspects of practice that students want and may need to understand (think through) and witnessed resuscitation is therefore a legitimate subject for contemplation and study.

Yet from the perspective of the standard model this topic is highly problematic. Putting to one side the not inconsiderable problems involved in disaggregating reason, motivation and value (Bond, 1983); the above questions, as phrased, might be considered unanswerable. Thus, regardless of how these informally framed queries are tidied up they will not be 'answered' by reviewing scientific research literature. Quantitative studies, for example, might tell us that some percentage of nurses, doctors, surviving patients and/or relatives do or do not think witnessed resuscitation should be allowed. And qualitative studies may advance claims about why particular nurses, doctors, etc., believe they think as they do. However, insofar as 'should' suggests the topic is being framed as an ethical/moral one – and it was always this aspect of witnessed resuscitation that interested students – then neither empiric quantitative nor qualitative research can resolve the issue.

In my experience, students invariably approach witnessed resuscitation normatively. And looked at in this way, it would not matter if quantitative research consistently found that 99.9% of people thought witnessed resuscitation a good or bad idea, if just one person thinks and argues that witnessed resuscitation should or should not be allowed on ethical/moral grounds, then that person is not wrong. Depending on what others say, we might conclude that their views are unpopular. Or, when articulated, we may take issue with the strength or persuasiveness of their argument. Yet insofar as the status of an ethical/moral belief is not a function of the number of people holding that belief, popularity or unpopularity is, in itself, immaterial. Put another way, counting rarely if ever resolves ethical/moral questions in a substantive or final sense.

Alternatively, it hardly matters which themes emerge in qualitative research. The self-reported 'feelings' or opinions of people favouring or dismissing witnessed resuscitation can be of interest. However, where qualitative findings reference emotions, then it must be conceded that the role of emotion in normative reasoning is difficult to assess. Indeed, while not my position (see also Mercier and Sperber, 2018), it might be claimed that emotion's role is, in this respect, irrelevant. For, while qualitative studies may establish that respondents hold certain views about a topic (perhaps passionately), and/or retrospective rationales for expressed views could be proposed, it is not unreasonable to suppose that psychology and emotion are largely extraneous to the analytic soundness of ethical/moral argument.

However, following comments in the Preface, we should be wary about unthinkingly separating reasoned argument from emotion. Thus, it could be objected that interests/bias inform or are informed by individual psychology and emotion, interests/bias cannot always be disaggregated from reasoning processes, and if this is granted, ethical and moral argument (reasoning) is or can be influenced by psychology/emotion. Nonetheless, descriptive statements about what 'is' (e.g. qualitative or quantitative findings) do not automatically support or map onto prescriptive statements about what 'ought' to occur and, the point stressed here, in addressing normative (evaluative) questions the primary appeal is – when justifications for positions are offered – to reason rather than research.

This does not mean research or what 'is' plays no part in deliberation. Yet in contradistinction to scientific inquiry, study findings support or challenge rather than lead non-scientific evaluative and normative thinking. And, crucially, values inform or commingle with reasoning in ways that, ideally, differ from the manner in which they permeate scientific inquiry. For example, a utilitarian inclined nurse reviewer could identify and scale (using research) the benefits and harms that attend witnessed resuscitation. And, informed by what is discovered, witnessed resuscitation might be favoured or rejected in some or all circumstances. However, significantly, it is the values informed theoretic position adopted that directs the choice and use of study findings. Alternatively, another nurse reviewer, perhaps taking a contrasting deontological stance, could read the same research and/or other findings, but reach diametrically opposed conclusions because their starting assumptions, their values and hence the trajectory through reasoning that they take, are different.

Of course, researchers also 'begin' with or cannot escape value bearing theoretic positions (articulated or not) and, for example, where radical forms of realism and constructionism oppose each other philosophically, studies following on from assumptions tied to these positions will be as influenced by the starting beliefs and values of researchers as are those noted above concerning evaluative and normative positions. (And I recognise that realism and constructionism themselves embody and rest on evaluative/normative assumptions.) Thus, in relation to ethical/moral questions, because utilitarians judge actions to be mandated or impermissible according to the results or consequences of those actions, and deontologists believe some actions are required or disallowed regardless of their results-consequences, different 'facts' (contrasting study findings) may be differentially important for utilitarians and deontologists. However, likewise, and equally crudely, because realists assume a real-world exists independently of observers, and constructionists hold that many or all of the real-world entities identified by realists are human constructions rather than mind independent entities; different 'facts' are potentially important for realist and constructionist researchers and, hence, grounded in these belief-value differences, different study findings can be concluded. This is granted.

Nevertheless, it is commonly (if disputably) supposed that science looks to external metrics (i.e. objective, observable, and reproducible measures) to resolve disagreement and where such metrics do not exist, neither does science.[2] If we wish to designate qualitative research as 'science' then, evidently, this definition problematises any such designation. However, side-stepping this difficulty, although normatively infused decisions can be informed and supported by scientific inquiry, because agreed metrics capable of adjudicating on the best or most appropriate ethical/moral stance to take in particular instances do not exist, questions that focus on or incorporate ethical/moral issues cannot be resolved where resolved implies provisional consensus can be derived using the measures stated above.

The word 'agreed' carries a great deal of weight in the preceding sentence. The meaning attached to the term demands unpicking, and this unpicking generates further devilishly tricky questions. Nonetheless, while (non-scientific) evaluative and normative inquiry cannot be settled in the same way that some (scientific) treatment option questions can be settled, this does not mean evaluative and normative questions are solely or solipsistically determined according to whimsical individual caprice. Rational people seek out pertinent facts (albeit that what counts as pertinent is contentious), and they consider and take into account the knowledge, beliefs, and opinions of others. Reviews dealing with evaluative and normative subjects can, when they bring in these considerations, make sense. And, thus, rather than 'simply' synthesising research findings (and there is nothing simple about synthesis), a nurse engaged with the problem of witnessed resuscitation might, for example, be expected to explain, compare and contrast a range of germane viewpoints *and* facts (both those they support and oppose), before or alongside outlining and arguing for the position they adopt. Moreover, adapting Chatfield (2017), it may be important that – however strongly certain views are held – reviewers ought to approach the literature in a manner that allows for the possibility that personal views might change (alter or be revised) consequent to being brought into contact with persuasive alternative arguments. However, to reiterate the point made earlier, from the perspective of the standard model and its attendant baggage, this is disastrous. Evaluative ethical/moral questions are necessarily 'bad' because they cannot be 'answered' (concluded) using research evidence.

In communion with others

Definitions of EBP note that alongside an up-to-date rationale (which is normally taken to mean research evidence), and the recognition of patient preferences, clinician judgement forms the third element in decision making (Ellis, 2016). However, few nursing studies meaningfully unpack what judgement involves, and subjectivity and subjective influence in decision making remains largely underexplored. Personally, I am not alarmed if decisions or, in the example used above (regards witnessed resuscitation), the conclusion of a literature review rely, in part at least, on non-empiric criteria. It is enough for me that a reviewer, having read widely and having considered what was read, has developed their thinking in a way that enables them to articulate and defend (at an appropriate level) their now extended thoughts on the subject in question. Yet, awkwardly, insofar as my institution strongly promotes use of CINAHL and kindred health orientated databases, and since specialist texts that might talk to evaluative and normative review questions in a substantive sense are infrequently located in these databases, students and researchers who follow taught search processes (mirroring the standard model) will be hard pressed to find what they need using the resources they are familiar with.

Further, marking criteria and module expectations presuppose use of something like the standard model when searches are conducted. And, to avoid disadvantaging students, whenever evaluative and/or normative questions of the type discussed here are raised, students may be warned about the difficulties they confront. In practice this means alternative answerable questions will probably be formulated (i.e. ones that address scientific rather than non-scientific and unanswerable problems). And, thus, 'Should witnessed resuscitation be allowed?' (an 'ought' query) becomes 'What percentage of nurses think witnessed resuscitation should be allowed?' (an 'is' query). This issue is revisited at various points throughout the book.

However, suffice to say, protecting students by closing down the subjects (here moral and/or ethical discourse) they engage with is distinctly unsatisfactory.

Hammering the point home, 'unanswerable' thus designates the improbability and/or impossibility of deriving fact-based consensus in certain circumstances. For example, circumstances in which evaluative and normative topics are considered. That said, scientific questions do not always generate consensus answers even when empiric evidence exists. And, further, regards moral questions, individuals can and do answer these to their own satisfaction when, often in communion and discussion with others, they develop or take up a stance in relation to specific questions. The phrase 'in communion … with others' is important here. I am persuaded to follow Hookway's (2013) reading of Peirce regards the significance of collective influences on individual deliberation albeit that confirmation bias and irrational 'group think' can and often does derail beneficial collective decision formation (Sloman and Fernbach, 2017). And, following on from this, when considering normative issues, the positions adopted by individual nurses need to be placed alongside the stance taken by nursing as a profession. Or, more accurately, the opinions of individual nurses can be informed by and contrasted against those expressed by other individuals and bodies who volunteer to speak for them.[3]

An imprecise label

Like 'non-scientific', 'unanswerable' is used here loosely. It is not a technical term. Nonetheless, despite its problematic nature, the phrase captures an important aspect or element of some questions addressed by nurses. That is, widespread unanimity or consensus is not always achieved or achievable in relation to evaluative and normative questions, nurses interest themselves in these questions, yet even when majority opinions form or are claimed to have been formed (i.e. when professional values are asserted), alternative minority positions and contradictory arguments are not necessarily wrong or incorrect in any formal sense, and to this extent, certain questions are unanswerable. Moreover, crucially, questions of this sort (e.g. normatively charged questions) are poorly served when procedures and ways of thinking more attuned to scientific questions are imposed upon them, and this, I suggest, occurs when commonly advanced search and review procedures (the standard model) inappropriately apply and enforce methodological norms and assumptions that were designed to meet scientifically grounded or closed questions. Nurses, like other healthcare professionals, rightly concern themselves with ethically laden and evaluative questions (e.g. 'what does compassionate care mean in this situation?'), and a great deal of student effort and published research explores this type of issue. This interest reflects the fact that nursing, like all human endeavour, is as much a normative enterprise as it is anything else. Yet research cannot, faced with these sorts of question, steer thinking or action in the same way that, it is supposed, some forms of, for example, quantitative research study can guide behaviour when purely technical or descriptive questions are addressed (e.g. *ceteris paribus* 'did more smokers quit smoking using new intervention 'x', rather than standard/old treatment 'y'?').

Positively, searches and reviews investigating evaluative and normative questions have value when they highlight and promote hitherto under or unexplored issues. These types of question are eminently worthy of consideration, they frequently stimulate or catalyse new ideas and fresh thought, and the positions we adopt and the arguments we accept in relation to this sort of discourse has as much potential to guide action as – by contrast – research findings. Further, while factual claims influence but do not determine evaluative and normative deliberation, evaluative and normative considerations likewise influence objective scientific research, as well as the uses to which science's products are put. However, to gain these benefits, to meaningfully get to grips with what evaluative and normative arguments have to offer, we need to rethink accepted ideas about what 'good' search and review practices encompass. And in this rethinking, and regardless of whether scientific or non-scientific questions are addressed, the importance of personal judgement and wide reading (i.e. reading within and also beyond nursing's traditional corpus) cannot be emphasised enough.

Beyond nursing – two cultures

The libertarian economist Murray Rothbard (2016 [1971]) thought that within his own domain of work "the quest for scientific truth" (p. 75), and the kudos that attaches to mathematical science, had encouraged the take up of distracting and stultifying practices. Worse, once established, scientific pretentions proved unamenable to revision. For, in the absence of external correctives (i.e. real-world objective metrics), when poor forms of reasoning take root in philosophy and social science, "it becomes much easier than in the physical sciences to ignore the existence of anomalies, and therefore easier to retain erroneous doctrines for a very long time" (ibid., p. 75). The erroneous doctrine that troubled Murray involved the triumphalism of particular forms of investigation, and as I understand him, an overemphasis on particular types of question. This produced changes in the reading practices of economists so that whereas: "Until recent decades, philosophers and social scientists harboured a healthy recognition of vast differences between their disciplines and the natural sciences … [and] the classics of philosophy, political theory, and economics were read not just for interest but for the truths that might lie therein" (ibid., p. 75), it is now assumed that, like the physical sciences, "all the contributions of past thinkers have been successfully incorporated into the latest edition of the currently popular textbook" (ibid., p. 76). And because "the disciplines of human action … [are now] frantically attempting to ape the methodology of the physical sciences … no one reads the classics in the field or indeed is familiar with the history of the discipline further back than this year's journal articles" (ibid., p. 76). Murray followed von Mises (1998) in situating economics as a discipline concerned with human action. He was aware that professionals act in the world, and the need for action guiding information was accepted. However, for Murray – like myself – this information (the ideas we might benefit from) is lodged within and across a variety of sources, these sources are not restricted to scientific outputs (vital those these are), and they are not 'owned' or controlled by a single profession or discipline. Indeed, while "the humanities and social sciences are increasingly expected to adopt the cultural norms of the hard sciences" (Macfarlane, 2017), these expectations should be resisted.

To raise the profile of what I take to be an underdiscussed issue, it has been proposed that nurses ask and concern themselves with scientific and non-scientific questions. Arguably this distinction is too prescriptive and/or simplistic. As presented the polarisation articulated excludes a middle way. That is, disciplines which bridge the gap are unrecognised and this does a disservice to, for example, social science, some branches of which welcome and allow questions that knowingly embrace and elide the answerable-unanswerable schism outlined here. It might therefore have been better to simply extol the benefits deriving from a liberal arts education (see e.g. Holmwood, 2011; Collini, 2012; Krislov, 2017). Or, alternatively and more ferociously, following Gray (2009 [1995]), the denigration of non-scientific questions that, in my view, the standard model of searching condones, could be placed within broader narratives of attack on enlightenment values.

Nevertheless, despite these qualifications the distinction being made has utility, and sticking with these descriptors, let us assume that questions seeking to answer scientific and non-scientific questions both have merit. Scientific questions may generate knowledge that, while fallible, provisional and contingent, is in principle obtainable using specified and agreed (generally experimental and objective) means. Alternatively, non-scientific questions address topics that, often, contain significant evaluative and normative components. These questions can illuminate thinking and inform action. However, the grounds on which this 'informing' is done vary dramatically from those underpinning the guidance offered by science. Non-scientific questions may be best approached using ideas and ways of thinking that emanate from or assume a humanities or arts heritage. And where this is the case, Snow's famous 'two cultures' 1959 Rede Lecture (1960) eloquently pointed towards the differences in thinking that distinguish each community.

Like Snow, we can grant that both forms of investigation have worth. However, since the standard model privileges scientific questions, and since education focuses on meeting the demands of this model, it might be supposed that nurses are undereducated and underprepared to address non-scientific questions with sufficient vim or rigour. A great deal of explanation will be required before nurses can establish how evaluative and normatively charged questions can best be pursued in literature reviews, and the use of humanity and arts-based resources is no less problematic for practitioners wishing to ground practice on 'evidence'. This book contributes to rather than concludes this discussion. Nonetheless, while there is nothing contentious in suggesting that scientific and non-scientific inquiry both have value, nurse writing presents a confused line on the place and usefulness of non-scientific endeavour and literary sources in nursing. Exacerbating this confusion, searches and reviews are – as noted in Chapter 1 – sometimes underappreciated in relation to all types of question.

Notes

1 Doctors often engage skilfully and subtly with non-biomedical subjects. Like nurses they are intimately concerned with patient- and family-centred care. Nonetheless, their education lays considerable stress on physical and medical science and it is this emphasis that is here accented.
2 Lord Kelvin's (William Thomson's) famous statement from *Popular Lectures* sums up key tenants of this viewpoint – thus: "I often say that when you can measure what you are speaking about, and express it in numbers, you know something about it; when you cannot express it in numbers, your knowledge is of a meagre and unsatisfactory kind; it may be the beginning of knowledge, but you have scarcely, in your thoughts, advanced to the stage of science, whatever the matter may be" (1883, p. 73–74).
3 The ability of corporate entities and groups (here nursing) to form, hold, and promulgate beliefs and/or values is, within the wider literature, debated and contested (see e.g. Hardin, 1982; Infantino, 1998; List and Pettit, 2011). Ontological and epistemological discussion on this subject lacks, however, a substantive foothold in nursing's literature – and perhaps because of this – a steady stream of commentators feel free to claim that, unproblematically, the totality of nurses jointly accept and maintain particular evaluative positions. That is, commentators frequently state that nurses believe or value any number of worthy things; and in using the collective 'nurses', we are presumably meant to take it that *all* nurses believe or value whatever is asserted. As the Preface notes, I baulk at such assertions. The claims advanced may be politically partisan. And because opinions differ it will in fact be the case that some (perhaps many) nurses reject views which, we are told, supposedly represent those espoused by 'the profession' in concert (Lipscomb, 2011; 2017b). That said, evaluative professional declarations cannot be ignored. They form an important facet of the 'communion ... with others' described here.

3

CONCEPTUAL MUDDLE

An ordinary search (part I)

- Fundamental concepts underpinning review processes lack clarity.
- Attention needs to be given to the wording of review purposes and questions.
- Relevance, comprehensive range, and partiality are problematised.

Chapter 2 proposed that nurses are concerned with, and ask, questions that might be labelled answerable-scientific and unanswerable-non-scientific. Hereafter, Chapters 3, 4 and 5 develop and expand upon this idea with reference to an example literature review. This example provides a frame around which problems of relevance, comprehensiveness and partiality are addressed. The example is loosely based upon – it stylises and adapts – work undertaken by a student I am familiar with. The review in question was done well, and the study it appeared in was praised. However, as will be shown, what we mean by 'good' is open to challenge. To maintain confidentiality, and to facilitate argument, the experience of this student is recast as a person henceforth known as pseudonymous Jane.

Statins and the media

Jane undertook a review into 'statins and the media'. Reading and reflection on experience led her to propose that the health risks accompanying statin use are sometimes misrepresented in the popular press. Specifically, they are overegged, and this distortion affects the way some patients interpret and act on, or fail to act on, medical and nursing advice. Tabloid misrepresentation of the balance of benefits and harms associated with statins can lead patients to refuse medication (Maksimainen, 2017; Nordestgaard, 2018) – and Jane, a GP practice nurse of many years standing, studied this issue in order that she could offer a countervailing correction. That is, part of alerting patients who have been prescribed statins to the importance of commencing and maintaining their use involves recognising and checking the malign influence and impact of press inaccuracy. To inform her understanding, a search was conducted.

Sequencing

Literature searches and reviews are goal directed and situated endeavours. Neither happens apart from the purpose for which it is performed or the context in which performance takes place. Indeed, regardless of the merits of any particular approach to location and appraisal, it is the confluence of purpose and context that determines (or should determine) where reviewers look, what they look for, and in large measure, how what is found is interpreted. Context carries several meanings in this book, and the connotations and significance of the concept is pursued across the next few chapters. Purpose, however, is no less fascinating. The term can be defined in a variety of ways, and the standard model's insistence that reviewers establish clear objectives before beginning a search represents one such characterisation. Put another way, every search (we are told) needs a purpose. It must be about something.

Sometimes this 'aboutness' is sharp, defined and succinct. In other instances, it is woollier. When a review's purpose is tightly bounded, fixed and demarcated, it may be possible to identify appropriate texts without undue drama. At other times ambiguity is present.

Questions bridge the gap between a review's purpose-objective and the literature. Occasionally, questions are synonymous with purpose-objectives. However, just as ambiguity can surround a review's purpose, when formulating questions, opacity is not uncommon. And, pointedly, once set, questions direct reviewer attention and behaviour. Explicitly, questions guide database and search term choices and, thereafter, what is located (normally research papers and systematic reviews of research papers) steer the form that analysis takes, the type of findings that are likely to be drawn, and the claims or recommendations that can be made on the basis of findings. How purposes and the questions that flow from them are worded is therefore of crucial importance. Sequencing matters.

Interpreting purpose

Wittingly or otherwise Jane was influenced in her search by the standard model. The model underpins teaching in the institution she studied at, and assumptions contained within it moulded aspects of her study. Her review, therefore, knowingly began by stating its purpose. That is, assuming the existence of the thing that interested her, Jane sought to appreciate the influence that media promulgated misinformation about statins exercises among or on a subgroup of patients prescribed this medication so that those misunderstandings could be managed and corrected. So far so good. Yet enunciating a review's purpose, defining the question or questions that need to be asked to meet that purpose, and picking keywords that identify papers pertinent to questions are not simple tasks. Problematically, purposes and the questions they spawn can often be articulated in more than one way, and as chapter one noted, apparently trivial differences in expression and interpretation (wording) may radically alter the path taken through location and appraisal. Indeed, numerous search 'trajectories' frequently exist for even straightforward purpose-questions.

Where reviewers explain and defend the decisions they take with regard to purpose, question, and search term choices, readers can take a view on whether sensible and rational choices were made. However, even when these sorts of issue are thought about, the type of detail being called for seldom appears in review write-ups. It can therefore be difficult to judge whether these aspects of the review process are done well. Indeed, it is unclear what 'doing well' means regards interpretation or wording.

Like Sherlock Holmes' 'dog that didn't bark',[1] this topic announces itself in silence. The overwhelming majority of published standalone reviews, supportive reviews, and student work (even that conducted at higher degree and doctoral level) disregard the possibility that different ways of framing purposes exist. Substantive reasons are rarely provided to justify the interpretations of purposes which are presented, and alternative readings are infrequently recognised. Similarly, review questions are generally stated in a manner that suggests the version chosen is the only one conceivable. Little or no explanation for particular question phrasings is given and, again, we are not told why rejected variants – alternative questions – are ignored. Nurse methodologists pay scant attention to this aspect of the review process. Yet where purposes can be differentially 'sliced and diced', and because judgements made at the outset of reviews about questions influence the direction of travel thereafter taken, this issue merits consideration.

While Jane recognised that the purpose of her review could be developed in several ways, these ways were not discussed in her report and no defence was offered to support the choices made. Inattention may partly be influenced by 'space'. That is, discussing these issues might require many hundreds of words, and given current norms around review practice, this sort of discussion could be seen as distracting or diversionary. Yet it is also the case that, even at higher degree level, educators do not normally prioritise or talk about these issues, journal editors do not insist that this topic is addressed and, hence, students and early career researchers cannot be blamed for overlooking them. I will shortly assert that, compared against others, Jane's was a good search. She certainly did nothing out of the ordinary. Nonetheless, although, for example, research on the topic of tabloid influence was located, her review did not focus exclusively on media related subjects. This was deliberate, but in the absence of explanation, readers of Jane's work may wonder why this line was taken.

Ambiguity matters because, in the form described (above), Jane's purpose-objective can be approached in several ways and, therefore, an explanation/defence needed to be offered in support of the version chosen. That is, clarification is necessary. For example, had the purpose been interpreted solely by reference to media reports, Jane might have looked at the media's power to influence opinion. And/or she might have mapped how newspapers portray statins. And/or good and bad examples of journalism could have been plotted. And/or temporal patterns in reporting might have been traced. And/or accuracy and balance across media outlets could have been compared and contrasted. Terms such as 'balance' throw up complex definitional problems. However, singularly or in concert each of these foci is consistent with the purpose of her review, and examining these subjects might have unearthed information of potential interest and benefit to patients and staff alike.

Alternatively, the review could simply have looked at why some patients give preferential credence to tabloid stories about statins over medical-nursing advice. This interpretation is as legitimate or warranted as those described above. Research on this topic was located. However, as per previous comments, this interpretation was not consistently tracked, and no reason for this was given. Had this approach been pursued then, as before, the review's purpose would have been interpreted in a particular manner. For example, expressing purpose in relation to 'credence' prompts exploration to take a psychological turn. The review might then have explored the literature on patient characteristics (attitudes, traits, dispositions, etc.) around or related to psychological 'dynamics' operative within a variety of scenarios (e.g. forms of nurse-patient interaction, the manufacture and maintenance of trust, or the nature and establishment of distrust).

Or, for the sake of argument, if we suppose interest settled on patient characteristics, studies from socio-behavioural psychology might have been sought examining patient responses to differently packaged advice. At a practical level, focusing on what patients do rather than why they act as they do, or say they act as they do, could usefully inform and direct written and verbal communication (among others Kahneman, 2012, is associated with the popularisation of this type of investigation). Research on this subject – psychological characteristics and the relationship between characteristics and behaviour – might be obtained through nursing, medical, or health related databases. However, it could and would probably be appropriate in this instance for analogous but apposite studies to be recruited from specialist psychological databases. Construing a review's purpose through a socio-behavioural lens here highlights the way in which a review's interpretation has implications for where searchers then go or look, as well as the skills that will be required by students/researchers in analysis (i.e. psychological research can utilise highly sophisticated forms of statistical test).

Then again, while still concerned with patient characteristics, the purpose might have been met by concentrating on cognitive functioning rather than behaviour. Thus, the review could have investigated whether patients who give credence to tabloid stories over medical-nursing advice differ in how they think about or process information compared with those taking contrary positions. Perhaps, for example, patients favouring tabloid sources have, on average, higher or lower educational qualifications than patients preferring medical-nursing advice. Or, feasibly, antagonism to medical-nursing advice might reflect the way in which, for example, negative attitudes to authority figures influence medical-nursing encounters. If research on either of these subjects was located it could help clinically situated nurses identify and target patients 'at risk' of underplaying the importance of medical-nursing guidance.

Note, it is not being suggested that a media *or* psychology emphasis should have been taken. There is nothing wrong in combining these and/or other approaches. Nor is it proposed that 'a' particular media or psychological interpretation of purpose is superior to another. Rather, it is argued that when or insofar as a review's purpose can be interpreted in more than one way – and these examples aim to demonstrate this possibility – reviewers should explain and justify the decisions they take regards interpretation. Each interpretation outlined here might lead to the location of evidence with clinical import. However, when reviewers do not adequately explain or defend their decisions (and remarkably few do), review readers confront two problems. They cannot judge whether sensible choices were made, and they will find it extremely difficult to assess the significance and potential importance of unexplored and overlooked options.

Objection

In response it might be objected that Jane's topic was overly vague from the outset and, therefore, it is hardly surprising that a varied array of purposes-objectives fall out of it. Perhaps if she had been more specific – if she had restricted her interests more carefully – the issues described above could be dissolved. For example, while this would mean abandoning the thing that intrigued her, had she focused attention instead simply on drug use/prescription, or an aspect of diagnosis/pathology, then a more 'controlled' review could have been structured.

Curtailing investigation to pathology would have enabled her to conduct a search using, for example, medical subject headings (MeSH) and in this way the presumptions of the standard model could be met and a 'tighter' review would ensue. However, while the arboreal and hierarchical structure of MeSH facilitates the swift retrieval of specific forms of published evidence, and although biomedical and non-biomedical MeSH descriptors exist,

MeSH searches limit the type of subject that can be explored. Indeed, while the U.S. National Library of Medicine has created a facility that greatly enhances the location of bio-medical literature, I can think of no good reason why nurses (or indeed anyone else) should restrict their inquiries to fit particular forms of search technology.

Further, even when appropriate – that is, when the use of MeSH would be helpful – it should be noted that very few nurses are trained to operate tools of this sort. Chapter 1 argued that if undergraduate students are not expected to read widely (i.e. locate and appraise anything other than a bare minimum of sources when constructing academic assignments), then we ought not to be surprised when post-graduates and early career researchers adopt similar attitudes/practices. In a kindred vein, even when post-graduate nursing students/ researchers are minded to perform rigorous searches, if undergraduate education has not sui-tably prepared them to do this, then given the time pressures and other demands made of post-graduates, the skills necessary to run complex reviews may not emerge. For a number of reasons, including the expressed desire to inculcate a sense of professional identify, under-graduates are frequently encouraged to treat CINAHL as their primary search engine. This approach does not preclude the use of supplementary engines. Nonetheless, insofar as CINAHL permits comparatively 'loose' keywords and phrases to be applied, and because undergraduates are not routinely required to engage with or utilise sophisticated engines – Jane – and I suspect a majority of post-graduate nursing students, would not, had it been suitable to do so, automatically have considered MeSH or OpenAthens or MedNets as potential resources (this list could clearly be extended).

Interpreting questions

Pivoting back to problems of justification, different conceptualisations of a review's purpose prompt different questions to be constructed and, once more, reviewers should explain why 'this' rather than 'that' formulation of a question is asked.

For example, had Jane focused on psychological matters, and had this interest been restricted to cognitive receptiveness and the relationship of receptiveness to trust, something akin to the following question might have been posed: 'Do patients who have experienced (in their view) prior negative medical-nursing encounters trust advice and information on statin use given by tabloid newspapers more than they trust information on this subject given by medical and nursing staff?' This is a tad wordy. Nevertheless, continuing the theme of interpretation, this type of question can be read in at least two ways, and this may be important.

Asking whether particular forms of prior experience differentiate between groups is the type of problem investigated by quantitative research. If a reviewer read the question in this way, phrases such as 'comparative study' would be fed into search engines and, surprise, quantitative studies will primarily be located. Yet, insofar as trust is an aspect of perception (and it is of course more than this), within the nursing literature (though not perhaps aca-demic psychological literatures), emphasising perception might encourage reviewers to employ search phrases such as 'patient experience', and in this instance, qualitative studies would be retrieved.[2] Alternatively, from the same starting point she could have asked: 'What number and/or percentage of patients offered statins preference media sources over medical-nursing advice in decision making?' The term 'preference' speaks to attitudes and dispositions. However, in contrast to the previous question, by explicitly referencing number, it is unli-kely that anything other than quantitative sources would be sourced.

Not only can 'a' review purpose be interpreted in more than one way, but 'an' interpretation of a purpose frequently generates multiple questions, and depending upon how these questions are worded, different search terms will be employed and different types of study will be identified. The questions outlined above are purely illustrative. Both address a formulation of the review's purpose, but each differentially sources qualitative and/or quantitative studies. Potentially, this difference impacts on the direction and conclusions that reviews take and reach. However, as with so many aspects of the review process, little discussion regards this issue takes place.

Synopsis

Questions about analysis reappear in this and subsequent chapters. Nonetheless, according to the standard model, before appraisal, purposes and questions must be set. On occasion this is an uncomplicated process. But, oftentimes, purposes and questions are open to interpretation. When this occurs, reviewers must make choices. Ideally – though this infrequently happens – these choices would be explained and defended, rejected choices would be described, and a rational for rejection given. Some details are provided in reviews and, for example, inclusion and exclusion criteria may be listed. Yet this hardly ever provides a meaningful explanation.

We should not, however, be overly hard on reviewers. After all, while purposes and questions must, it is asserted, be formulated before a review is conducted, counterintuitively, the results of the review being undertaken might be needed to rationally set these things in the first place. Put another way those making decisions may, at the beginning of the process, be operating 'in the dark'.

The standard model and almost all methodologists thus require that reviewers start by establishing clear purposes and questions. The precise wordings of these determine what is located. What is located steers the conclusions that can be drawn, and – if such be the aim – any recommendations for practice/research that are made. However, the knowledge required to rationally make decisions might not, in advance of the review being undertaken, be available. (Note, I am not here invoking Meno's paradox or the paradox of inquiry.) Heuristic organising tools (e.g. CMO or CIMO, ECLIPS(E), PICO or PICOT or PICOTT, SPICE, SPIDER, etc.) exist to help reviewers structure their thinking (Davies, 2011; Methley et al., 2014). Yet, while the value of these devices should not be underestimated (particularly when systematic reviews are being planned – Saimbert, Pierce and Hargwood, 2017), they could, on occasion, be accused of enabling reviewers to offer spurious justifications for decision making. That is, although these sorts of device reveal something of the reasoning involved in framing purposes and questions, from a reader's perspective, they are often less than enlightening. Like inclusion and exclusion criteria (Chapter 1), lists generated by these tools often add little to understanding. Well intentioned commentaries on the use of these devices oversimplify the issues involved (see e.g. Khodabux, 2016) and – indeed – it is perhaps a mistake to suppose that 'correct' ways of proceeding exist.

Alternatively, it could be objected that too great an emphasis is being placed on the difference between purposes and questions. After all, overlap between these two things is large and, often, they are (or come close to being) synonymous.[3] Maybe. However, choices around purpose, question and search term wording are rarely clarified or defended in a meaningful or non-superficial sense. Many reasons for this exist. Most 'how to' guides tend not to explore these sorts of issue and, perhaps, recognising these problems undercuts the sort of bullish certainty that is assumed in methodological texts. By this I mean, review methodologies tend to embody or present a declamatory notion of structure that would be destabilised if the uncertainties thrown out by worries around wording and interpretation were realised. This is speculation. Nonetheless, reviewers take important 'steering' decisions at the start of reviews on the basis of not much evidence and, hence, these decisions can be difficult to justify. Framing purposes, deciding on the wording of questions, and choosing search terms are delicate matters. Minor changes in phrasing can redirect emphasis and, therefore, the results obtained. Information that would enable choices to be made on logical or defendable grounds may only be available after a review is concluded and, by then, it is too late.

Interpreting scope

The scope of a review must also be established at the outset and, again, this involves choices. Jane had the option of focusing narrowly on nursing, medical and health related literatures, or she could formulate purposes and questions more broadly. That is, she could expand the subject of inquiry to bring in non-nursing and non-health literatures. Curiously, this facet of the review process often passes unnoticed and key decisions are frequently made by default. Thus, the standard model, as interpreted in nursing, pushes reviewers to use nursing and medical-health orientated databases and websites (e.g. CINAHL plus, perhaps, Medline, etc.), and because of this, reviewers may not deliberately or overtly decide upon scope. Instead, following norms built into the standard model, they may unwittingly ask 'What do nursing and medical-health related databases say is known or believed about "x" ?', rather than 'What is known or believed about "x"?' And, clearly, these are or can be very different things. (Here and elsewhere I follow Wilson, 1967, in differentiating between knowing and believing.)

The approach taken by Jane is described below. However, like the majority of postgraduate students/researchers, in addition to failing to explain or defend the interpretations of purpose and question wording used in her review (where the purpose and questions it gave rise to were collapsed into each other), and on top of failing to mention alterative interpretations and/or phrasings for purposes and questions, she did not meaningfully look outside of nursing and health related literatures. Additional sources were accessed. Yet her investigation of non-nursing and non-health related material remained fairly superficial. Mainly, her search stuck to CINAHL and Medline, and the review was comparatively narrow in scope.

That said, because nurses turn to the literature to inform nursing practice, some authorities' actively sanction or promote the adoption of a constricted approach. Clearly review purpose-questions steer investigations, and if purpose-questions can be satisfactorily resolved by focusing only on nursing material, then nursing databases should be targeted. 'Satisfactory' is somewhat question begging. However, this aside, some questions (e.g. 'What does nursing research say about "x"?') can be addressed through discipline specific sources, whilst others (e.g. 'What are appropriate treatments for patients diagnosed with "x"?') may require that nursing and medical-health related sites be investigated (that said, see previous comments regards MeSH).

Thus, when review purpose-questions address scientific or treatment option problems that are described in nursing, medical, and health literatures, it may be unnecessary to look elsewhere. However, when non-scientific topics and unanswerable questions are investigated, and when action based upon the findings of scientific investigation is being considered, a wider range of materials should potentially be reviewed. Contra both the standard model and those who wish to limit the remit of nurse interests, it can be and often is sensible for reviewers who take up anything other than a very tight group of scientific ('closed') problems to look beyond health-related sources. This claim is based on an expanded notion of relevance (discussed shortly) and the 'beyond' referred to here includes, or can include, humanities and arts texts. In this more open approach to searching, deterministically linking purposes to questions, to what is located, to the form that appraisal takes, to the findings and conclusions that are drawn, may be refused albeit that, ultimately, whether a narrow or broad approach to reviews is pursued is a matter for argument rather than assumption or dictat.

This said, and as previously noted, too much may be being read into the setting of purpose-questions and the establishment of scope. Experienced reviewers adapt search strategies to meet their needs, and while nurse methodologists appear reluctant to engage with the 'wording issues' detailed above, alternatives to the standard model are, to repeat, lodged in the better methodological texts. Yet, caveats aside, students and early career researchers who rely on these texts for guidance will find themselves obliged to set purpose-objectives, questions, and 'scope' (and establish search terms, and chose databases etc.) before reviews commence. And new or raw reviewers may mechanistically and obediently follow standard model strictures even when this is not sensible. Subsequent chapters outline the case for recognising and promoting evolving searcher interests over standard model demands, it is proposed that the pre-eminence given to 'methods' can sometimes be upended or overturned, and it is not the case that reviewer interests and concerns must always be sublimated to 'process'. However, before this case is made, other elements of conceptual disorder demand recognition.

Conceptual disorder

Students and novice researchers look to methodological texts for guidance. Yet, when simple and complex review procedures are described, either a lot is left unsaid, or what is said is hard to digest. Parahoo (2006), for example, states that supportive reviews are undertaken "to inform" (p. 121) projects and contextualise knowledge. This makes sense. However, the nature of 'informing' is left hanging. The concept is vague. Does 'to inform' mean that all, most, many, or some appropriate sources were accessed and digested? Does the phrase reference a psychological state (e.g. the reviewer now feels informed), or does it ground an epistemological claim (e.g. a quantity of knowledge now informs)? I presume the latter. But what does a quantity of informing look like? Similarly, while Booth, Papaioannou and Sutton (2012) ask reviewers to pay special attention to "more nuanced findings" (p. 136), this is simply question begging. How are nuanced findings being identified? Where is the nuanced-unnuanced demarcation line drawn? What non-tautologous metric is being applied in decision making? And, while Coughlan and Cronin (2017) sensibly warn reviewers not to include "irrelevant publications" (p. 69) and sources which are "interesting" (p. 69) but that do not address "your question" (p. 69) – and who would disagree? – without explaining how relevance and pertinence are being established, these cautions serve little use.

Mercier and Sperber (2018) note that "a logical demonstration can never be stronger than its weakest part" (p. 21) – and insofar as they attempt to make clear or establish knowledge/understanding in relation to a purpose-question, reviews can be thought of as demonstrations. However, while methodological texts vary in sophistication, regardless of erudition and/or the complexity of argument, they rarely provide readers with the detail needed to make sense of or evaluate what is said. This important issue was hinted at in chapter two.

Nonetheless, methodological ambiguity of this sort threatens to undercut the strength of review 'demonstrations' and, for example, Aveyard, Payne and Preston (2016) provide an explanation of meta-ethnography (an interpretive approach to reviewing qualitative studies) that largely skirts over what is involved.

Helpfully (or not), readers are told that meta-ethnography is "not for the novice" (ibid., p. 26), and this should put most people off investigating further. However, claims that "you aim to explore concepts in detail rather than simply report and summarise the findings of a range of studies" (ibid., p. 26) are, even with the provision of an example, difficult to understand. What, for example, does 'exploring concepts in detail' involve? How much detail is required? What is 'a range', and how big should it be? The readers of methodological texts are unlikely to know what these sorts of injunction mean. On the other hand, it is quite reasonable to expect that reviewers wishing to use approaches they are unfamiliar with will seek out specialist instruction. This presumes naïve readers can, on the basis of limited information, realise that they might or should adopt an approach that differs from the standard model. Yet this aside, reading back into primary sources can, unfortunately, add to rather than ameliorate confusion.

Aveyard, Payne and Preston (2016) reference Noblit and Hare (1988) in describing meta-ethnography. However, Noblit and Hare do not write for novices. Their thinking instead aims to stimulate discussion as well as explain, and the reference provided by Aveyard, Payne and Preston (2016) does not then identify a beginner's 'how to' guide. Positively, Noblit and Hare (1988) propose that meta-ethnography prizes interpretation over aggregation. This I like. They also kick back against excessive explicitness and bureaucratisation (i.e. over processual forms of review-analysis). Again, this is attractive. Moreover, their claim that "synthesis reveals as much about the perspective of the synthesizer as it does about the substance of the synthesis" (ibid., p. 14), is one that resonates with me (see Preface). Yet in their embrace and use of metaphor, Noblit and Hare present a way of conducting reviews that runs counter to the thrust of other claims in Aveyard, Payne and Preston (2016). Specifically, Noblit and Hare (1988) allow greater scope or rein to imaginative interpretation than the more literalist approach found in Aveyard, Payne and Preston (2016), and this is problematic on two counts.

First, readers who rely on Aveyard, Payne and Preston (2016) for their understanding of meta-ethnography are not given the detail they need to make sense of and employ the approach on offer. Second, readers who turn to Noblit and Hare (1988) will confront an interesting and thought-provoking approach to reviewing that jars when set alongside other more formulaic review processes described by Aveyard, Payne and Preston (2016). This sort of disjuncture can be found throughout nurse methodological writing.

Judgment and relevance

The standard model dominates practice. However, methodological texts define and juxtapose approaches to location and appraisal that are mutually contradictory or inconsistent. These contrasting approaches often differ markedly and, moreover, the description of important concepts is regularly fudged.

Conceptual muddle in the methodological literature is a significant issue. And, arguably, the absence of clarity is most pressingly felt in regard to 'relevance'. Like everyone else, Jane sought to locate relevant rather than irrelevant sources in her review. However, determining the nature of this thing and knowing when relevance is achieved is no easy task. The descriptor is, in methodological writing, ubiquitous. Yet although something of its meaning can be gleaned from the manner in which it is presented, this pervasive and vital concept is rarely explained in anything other than abstractly sweeping terms. Sticking with non-committal abstractness, relevance, for me, exists in the intersection between what is asked, and what is deemed appropriate in answering or addressing what is asked. Some sources are, in context, self-evidently relevant. Others are not. However, since relevance does not identify itself, *someone* must establish or claim to establish this thing. And this aspect of the concept – its reliance on human judgement – is underappreciated and underdeveloped in the majority of methodological texts that nurses encounter.

The question – how can reviewers judge and justify claims for relevance? – is tackled shortly. Here I focus on a different but allied question, namely, how much of what is relevant must be found? Or, put another way, what can be omitted? Superficially these last questions reframe those asked by the student in chapter one (i.e. 'What's the smallest number of papers I need to review?'). There, the idea that a set number of papers could sensibly be identified for location in advance of appraisal taking place was ridiculed. That criticism stands. However, these questions here provide a jumping off point in the opening gambit of an argument favouring a more expansive approach to reading (i.e. one that allows questions to be 'addressed' as well as 'answered'). This manoeuvre rests on the notion that unanswerable or non-scientific questions (as defined in chapter two) can and sometimes should be explored. It also permits an approach to searching for and reviewing literature to be developed that gives due prominence to the evolving interests of those involved. And, as will be shown, introducing the concept of personal interests permits the questions we ask to play a crucial and different role in location and appraisal to those which are usually allotted to them.

Comprehensive and reasonable

Jane's concern with a particular form of professional-patient interaction might, as stated, have been articulated in several ways. Further, and again as described, regards scope, she chose to treat the topic relatively narrowly. Thus, research papers and to a lesser extent systematic reviews and official guidelines were primarily targeted. However, she also sought out a limited number of non-nursing and non-research sources (e.g. media reports misconstruing statin use), and relevance was therefore not reduced entirely to a reading of nursing and health related papers. That said, the approach taken largely reflected taught practice (the standard model) and Jane's search strategy was influenced by Aveyard, Payne and Preston's (2016) *A Post-graduate's Guide to Doing a Literature Review*. This work (previously cited) is squarely aimed at advanced students and researchers. It is suggested reading at the institution Jane studied at (for students operating at her level).

Aveyard, Payne and Preston (2016) assert that reviewers usually aim "to identify all of the published and sometimes unpublished literature that relates to your review question" (p. x). This claim is unambiguous, bold, and insofar as 'all' recognises no limits, it is unboundedly aspiring. Aveyard, Payne and Preston (2016) go on to caveat and contradict this statement. Nevertheless, calls to locate 'all' or a 'comprehensive range' of relevant literature that 'relates to your review' are regularly repeated in texts that students and researchers encounter. For example, Punch (2005, p. 266), Coughlan and Cronin (2017, p. 2) and Moule (2018, p. 57) stress the importance of accessing a "comprehensive" range. Booth, Papaioannou and Sutton

(2012) emphasise the need for reviewers to access "all" relevant sources (p. 3), and Aveyard (2018) defines reviews as overviews "of all research undertaken in a particular area" (p. 4).

A sizeable number of papers (approx. 50) were located in Jane's search, and if the quantity of retrieved materials had to be described, the phrase 'very reasonable' could easily be applied. Indeed, while I did not grade her work, had I done so, I would have commented favourably on the volume of sources located. Yet, bar approval, it is not clear what this compliment conveys. As an educator and journal reviewer I look, among other things, at how many papers are cited in student essays and submitted reports. Generally speaking, the use to which citations are put is considerably more important than the sheer quantity of names listed. That is, we want writers to employ relevant citations to support and advance argument and merely cataloguing who said what is, by and large, less vital (Thompson, 2017). Nonetheless, employed appropriately, I expect to see a judicious number of citations. Yet, how many is enough? What is reasonable? What is judicious?

Unsurprisingly, 'reasonable' is a tricky word to define, and this lack of specificity lends it a weaselly quality. With regard to Jane's study, reasonable references a number commensurate with the achievements of similarly placed students/researchers undertaking comparable work at the institution she studied at. However, other institutions employ different norms regards such matters, and local expectations are somewhat arbitrary. Further, no necessary link exists between citing a 'reasonable' and 'comprehensive range' of sources. That is, citing a reasonable number against local expectations, and citing a comprehensive range of relevant sources, can be and probably are entirely different things.

Comprehensiveness and partiality

Given the scope and nature of the topic under investigation it could be claimed that, inevitably, relevant texts will have been overlooked by Jane's search (later chapters suggest this is what happened) and, perhaps, accessing a 'reasonable number' is the best that can be hoped for. Maybe – but – if 'all' sources were not recovered, and if the lesser descriptor 'comprehensive range' cannot be shown to have been achieved, then the findings or outcomes of her search reflect a partial reading of the literature and, presumably, partial readings are necessarily less informative and useful than non-partial ones. Potentially, partial readings can distort rather than illuminate understanding.

Associating the idea of distortion with partiality is problematic when or insofar as it suggests these readings fail against a hypothetical or imagined non-distorted analysis of all or a comprehensive range of objectively determined relevant papers. This convoluted statement requires unpacking. And this notion of distortion is critiqued in Chapter 5. However, here I want to stress that, although the extent and impact of partiality cannot easily be quantified, it may be that the majority of searches locate and analyse only a fraction of available applicable and informative (i.e. relevant) material.

The importance of partiality presumably varies. Sometimes it will matter a lot that only a fraction of relevant sources are located and assessed. For example, a well-resourced review conducted with the intention of establishing how patient care can be improved should not evidence excessive partiality since this conceivably compromises its usefulness. Alternatively, at other times failure matters less. For example, a first-year undergraduate student essay performed to practice search skills is not expected to meet the methodological standards attained by experienced and skilled analysts. Nevertheless, regardless of partiality's effect, like 'reasonable', 'comprehensive range' (in many ways the flip side of partiality) lacks a sub-stantive or agreed meaning, and it is often therefore impossible to determine if or when this range is achieved.

Thus, although we can determine when a search is demonstrably partial (i.e. by identifying the absence of key texts we might be able to justifiably assert that a comprehensive range of available relevant literature has not been located), even when searchers access exceptional quantities of high quality relevant sources, because the descriptor 'comprehensive' does not have a settled denotation, it can be difficult to categorically state that a search deserves this title. Moreover, given the prominence allotted to the term by methodological writers, defi-nitional vagueness regarding the concept is perplexing.

How then is comprehensive to be comprehended? The word might be understood in relation to the breath or scope of a search. That is, comprehensiveness could be a function of the narrowness and/or broadness of a review. Thus, had Jane only wanted to ascertain whether the nursing literature recognised media influence as a problem vis-à-vis statin use, she could have combed CINAHL using comparatively tightly defined search criteria. It is conceivable that all, or nearly all, relevant sources might be located in this way and given this possibility few or no excuses could have been made had a comprehensive range not been located. Alternatively, had her inquiry sought to understand the topic broadly, comprehen-siveness may be more difficult to achieve or demonstrate. For example, had her interest set-tled on why some patients prefer media over medical-nursing information sources, she might have set questions on (among other things) past experience as an influencing factor in trust formation (as discussed). That is, she could have explored whether patients who believe previous medical-nursing information and advice was wrong or unhelpful are steered towards or more likely to prefer 'trusted' media sources over 'untrusted' medical-nursing ones. Had this route been taken, while some pertinent material would be located in nursing-health databases, non-nursing and non-health sites might also be considered appropriate. And in opening up the range of sites and sources thought suitable, while a wider range of sources would be accessed (and a clearer overall picture might be gained), the partiality of her search would presumably increase as comprehensiveness declines. Thus – awkwardly – if we define a good search as one that allows reviewers to grasp or gain a reasonable overview of what is known and believed (i.e. if a good search maximises learning), then potentially at least this better view comes at the cost of increased partiality and reduced comprehensiveness.

The point here is that although relevance, and hence partiality-comprehensiveness, are functions of what is asked and what is believed to be appropriate, comprehensiveness can be maximised when questions are set in ways that, for example, require only limited subsets of nursing literature to be reviewed. Cynically, it might be wondered whether the desire to control the number of sources located lies behind methodological advice promoting narrowly defined questions. However, problematically, setting narrow questions (for whatever reason) may prove unproductive. That is, narrowly defined questions might not facilitate searches that locate sources capable of maximally improving patient care and/or progressing research concerns. Thus, while the interests of those performing reviews determine relevance, searches that are too narrow may miss important information and insights and, also, the standard model's requirement that only particular literatures and/or sources be accessed is similarly outlandish.

Representativeness and comprehensive range

Before charging on, a common misconception must be laid to rest. Namely, in the absence of 'all' papers it might be assumed (mistakenly) that 'comprehensive range' references representativeness. That is, it might be imagined that comprehensiveness stands for or is achieved when a representative sample of available relevant literature is located.

> If ... your final intention is to sample judiciously from the literature ... then you need to have confidence that your sampling frame has been constructed appropriately.
>
> *(Booth, Papaioannou and Sutton, 2012, p. 136)*

Phrases such as 'sample judiciously' and 'sampling frame' can, in the quotation above, be read in several ways. Nonetheless, language of this sort might suggest that a comprehensive range is achieved or located when a sufficient *sample* of sources are identified. I could be misrepresenting Booth, Papaioannou and Sutton (2012). However, they approvingly cite Atkins et al. (2008) who also refer to establishing populations of studies from which to sample, and this type of language is widely identifiable. Thus, it appears some methodologists think that a sample representative of the findings and/or arguments and ideas located in all relevant literature might be identified. And, in addition, I have heard lecturers say similar things to students. Two closely related versions of this line of reasoning can be described. Neither holds water.

First, if an agreed percentage of relevant papers could be accessed from the total pool available, then against this measure, it might be claimed that a comprehensive range was retrieved. For example, if an agreed percentage of all relevant papers were located, and if this percentage met or exceeded a statistically determined threshold, it could be supposed that good reason exists to confidently predict that a representative selection or sample of findings, arguments and ideas have been located. Second, it may be suggested that we should seek to identify an agreed percentage of all papers, again against a statistically agreed standard, that meet some sort of quality-relevance criteria. Thus, within the set of all relevant papers, we might look for an agreed percentage, a sampled subgroup, of high-quality papers. For either option to obtain it would be necessary to establish the totality of relevant sources available (in which case why not simply access and review them?), as well as, in the later scenario, the quality of all pertinent papers.

The idea that it is possible to locate all or almost all relevant papers in anything other than a tiny number of specific cases is, as suggested, ambitious. In these 'cases' very tightly defined scientific and/or treatment option questions must be asked, and only a small number of known sources should relate to that option. Moreover, even then, it might be argued that inclusion-exclusion criteria are too narrowly drawn and, thus, simply because scientific and/or treatment option (answerable) questions can be defined in a manner that limits what is found, this does not mean they should be so defined. Further, in many and possibly most instances, reviewers will not know what 'all' relevant papers reference and, thus, this element of the representativeness-comprehensiveness association can be parked.

On the other hand, quality is considered by searchers. Studies of 'good' quality are sought, and poorly conducted studies are removed from analysis. Poor quality studies are excluded because their findings are not trusted. Poor quality here refers to conduct (i.e. how a study is performed), and it is assumed that where unreliable processes of knowledge creation are used, discoveries lack credibility. In Chapter 5, the concept of epistemic reliabilism is introduced. This concept emphasises the importance of belief forming processes (tokens) in establishing confidence in knowledge claims, and it is the absence of this element of research design and execution that 'poor quality', in this context, identifies. Epistemic reliabilism is a perfectly respectable theory. However, it is not the only contender in this field, and when we look at research, significant disagreement surrounds the meaning and nature of 'good' and 'bad' methods. Reviewers therefore need to be wary when differentiating between studies on the basis of quality. Clearly, good and bad quality research exists, and excluding poor quality studies from reviews makes sense. Yet, the criteria against which quality is assessed should be described and justified and, inevitably, alternative perspectives are available. Determining quality is rarely straightforward.

For example, reviewers looking at quantitative evidence may privilege generalisable over less generalisable studies if or when better generalisability is associated with better quality. That is, generalisability and quality can be and often are elided. This assumption stimulates comparatively little interest in nursing methodological texts. However, not only is it open to dispute (see e.g. Pawson, 2006), but practically establishing generalisability at the level of an individual study is both complex and complicated. Reviewers relying on quantitative material can reasonably presume that a well-conducted randomised controlled trial potentially produces more generalisable results than a well-conducted non-experimental study. Nonetheless, this claim has been problematised and challenged (Bluhm, 2016; Kerry, 2017; Krauss, 2018), and even if accepted, sophisticated skills are required before the findings of 'this' as opposed to 'that' randomised trial can be deemed more or less generalisable. Further, since randomised trials vary across a number of parameters (including generalisability), unless reviewers treat all trial results as being equally generalisable (which they are not), detailed assessment is necessary. Confidence intervals and other statistical devices assist assessment and generalisability is, within parameters, measurable. Yet using and checking that tests are accurately performed is no simple matter, and it is not at all evident that nurse students and researchers possess the skills required to carry out this form of scrutiny (chapter six develops this argument).

Regards qualitative research, while these studies can unlock hitherto unrealised ideas and ways of looking at the world, this type of research cannot, according to traditional scientific thinking, produce generalizable findings (Niaz, 2007; Janardhana et al., 2018). This claim is disputed (Lewis and Ritchie, 2003; Polit and Beck, 2010; Smith, 2018). Nevertheless, the inclusion of qualitative studies in reviews raises a host of thorny issues and their clinical applicability is difficult to assess (Malterud, 2001; Golafshani, 2003; Shenton, 2004). Thus, while a vast range of evaluative guides are proposed (see e.g. Probyn, Howarth and Maz, 2016; Santiago-Delefosse et al., 2016), agreed standards for judging the quality of qualitative research do not exist (Leung, 2015), and significant doubts about the theoretical robustness of published qualitative studies have been raised (Lau and Traulsen, 2017). Chapter 7 explores this issue in more detail.

For both qualitative and quantitative research (let alone other evidence sources) pragmatic and other difficulties 'complicate' and may indeed prevent the quality of sources from being established. Where this occurs, postulated links between quality and comprehensiveness are severed, and in anything other than unusual circumstances, it is thus foolhardy to tie 'comprehensive range' to both representativeness as a percentage of all relevant papers, and/or representativeness as a percentage of good quality relevant papers. Alternatively, if comprehensive references a dimension of representativeness (and I do not think it does), then perhaps the relationship pertains in some way to a mixed bag or spread of material being accessed. That is, describing a search as comprehensive could signal that a representative range of different forms of relevant evidence have been located-assessed.

As stated, Jane's search accessed research papers and to a lesser extent, systematic reviews, guidelines, and, also, a smattering of illustrative commentaries including newspaper and magazine stories. Given the theme of her enquiry, it was probably necessary that this variety of material be located. Yet if comprehensiveness refers to the location of a mixed bag or spread of materials, do the same number of each type of source need to be found? Or, as occurred, are some sources (e.g. primary research reports) more valued or valuable than others (e.g. commentaries)? Fundamentally, how, in any inquiry, can different types of evidence be weighted in importance or relevance and what, if any, relationship does relevance have to notions of comprehensiveness as representativeness?

It might be supposed that the hierarchy of evidence could be used as a tool through which these questions can be addressed, and if generalisability was the only criterion against which comprehensiveness and relevance were being judged, it may be plausible that sources from the apex of this hierarchy meet the weighting problem identified here. Yet, depending on the purpose-question being addressed, generalisability is unlikely to be the only factor 'in play'. The hierarchy or hierarchies (multiple versions of this thing exist) downgrades and largely ignores qualitative and non-research sources, and in some instances, non-research sources might well be the ones we are most interested in.

Reprise

Asking these questions hopefully illustrates their silliness. It is clearly nonsensical to propose that weightings for different types of literature can or should be set, and while partiality can be linked to potential unrepresentativeness, I do not believe comprehensiveness requires representativeness. However, since Aveyard (2018), like others, defines reviews as research (described Chapter 1), and since representative samples are important features of quantitative research (and quantitative biases inform the standard model), this association must be confronted.

The problem is – to end where we began – there is no meaningful or substantive consensus on what relevance means. Moreover, even if consensus existed on what relevance was (and this would require additional agreements on the precise wording of purpose-questions), since in most instances we are unlikely to locate all relevant papers on a topic, reviewers must concern themselves with the slippery concepts of 'comprehensive range' and 'partiality'.

Methodologists have a great deal of work yet to do in resolving these concepts. And, for example, Parahoo (2006), who offers one of the best short guides to research, is as elusive as everyone else on the meaning of relevance. Thus, while researchers should review an array of "up-to-date, relevant and credible" (p. 126) sources, when it comes to scope we are told that "The researcher should cast her net wide in order to 'feel the pulse' of the phenomenon she is studying" (p. 126). Parahoo does not exaggerate the significance of research reports among the materials that are to be located. However, as guidance, 'feeling the pulse' is, in relation to relevance, an evocative but possibly unhelpful phrase. Researchers who turn to this work hoping for clarification are told that searches and reviews are conducted "to put the current study into the context of what is known already" (p. 127). That contextualisation allows comparisons to be made across "similar studies" (ibid., p. 128), and that "It is not important or necessary to discuss every previous research study in detail (ibid., p. 131). These claims are sensible and systematising processes that restrict flexibility should be rejected. Nonetheless, this is all quite hazy. Questions tumble out from these sorts of statement and, for example, what does 'putting into context' require? How many relevant papers must be read to enable this laudable goal? And, again, what is relevant? How is context to be determined or evaluated? How alike must similar studies be for realistic comparisons to be made? Since no two studies are identical, at what point does dissimilarity make comparison unfeasible? How is this point to be established? And if it is not necessary to discuss every previous (relevant?) study, how are inclusion-exclusion decisions being made? How will they be justified?

Parahoo (2006) does meet this last query insofar as the need to argue a case through presented materials is emphasised. Yet, the point being stressed, even the best of guides leaves bedrock questions untouched and unanswered.

Notes

1 *The Adventure of Silver Blaze* – Arthur Conan Doyle (2018 [1892]).
2 Experience in this second example references psychological experience rather than, as in the first example, perceived events in the world (experience of the world). Obviously, both forms of experience 'overlap' and commingle. However, they also come apart. Psychological experience can refer to mental happenings such as emotional states which take place 'within' the experiencing organism, while 'in the world' signals – or can signal – experience (as event representations) of mind independent happenings. Experience like perception is not then a simple term. It carries multiple meanings and it is used in various ways. Failure to note these ways generates much confusion.
3 That search questions can differ from the stated purpose of a study may strike some as odd. However, first, as argued, following standard model precepts, review purposes are interpreted through the questions they give rise to and – allied to this – second, research aims and objectives frequently generate or are articulated in purposes and questions that, to be addressed coherently, require reviewers to look 'beyond' particular purposes/questions.

4

BELIEFS AND VALUES

An ordinary search (part II)

- Definitional imprecision is explored further.
- Performing reviews systematically does not overcome identified difficulties.
- The role of beliefs and values in location and appraisal are outlined.
- The significance of judgement in review processes is reasserted.
- A potentially positive role for non-research and non-nursing texts in reviews is claimed.

Against local expectations (i.e. institutional standards and norms) Jane's search might, as noted, be judged good, and her work was favourably received. Yet the review, which was quite narrowly constrained (see Chapter 3), accessed an unknown percentage of available sources, of variable quality, from across a constricted range of evidence types. The wisdom of linking relevance with sampled percentages of sources has been discussed and dismissed. Nevertheless, it is possible to identify pertinent overlooked texts (discussed in Chapter 5), and stating that an unknown percentage of relevant sources were retrieved highlights the partial nature of her search. Moreover, beyond contingent and ad hoc local norms, because there are no agreed or objective means of establishing when comprehensiveness is achieved, one of the few things we can say for certain about the search is that if key ideas and arguments located within the wider literature were retrieved, this achievement occurred by chance rather than design. At root, since we do not know the extent of partiality, we do not know how unrepresentative and possibly skewed (or not) located information was.

Thinking, belief, knowledge, action

Reading stimulates thinking and, put crudely, thinking affects what is believed and known (or thought to be known). Further, although the links, mechanisms and relationships between thinking and doing are notoriously fuzzy and ill-defined, belief and knowledge influence action/behaviour in some if not all instances. Material sourced in her search is likely to have informed Jane's beliefs and knowledge. And potentially at least, 'informed' belief and knowledge will alter aspects of her future interactions with patients. However, because, presumably, action/behaviour in a clinical environment should not knowingly rest or be grounded on partial and incomplete information, since we cannot accurately assess or determine comprehensiveness, and since hers was a partial search, it could be concluded that the evidence and ideas gleaned ought not to inform practice.

These statements can be criticised and, for example, the things we believe and know (think we know) are affected by all sorts of half-baked ideas, ill-considered forms of reasoning, and dodgy data. It is thus unreasonable to propose that action based on belief-knowledge will not utilise screwy mental processes and factual inaccuracies. Moreover, while it is sensible to presume that beliefs and knowledge should rest on epistemically good rather than bad grounds, this is a relative claim. Partial information – even markedly partial information – may, in some instances, be better than no information. And to complicate matters, good reasons exist for knowingly acting on poor information. For example, we should perhaps act on weak epistemological grounds when the risk associated with not acting is great and the burden or cost of acting is low. Thus, if someone yells 'Fire' consider leaving where you are even if you cannot see smoke/flames, or smell burning, and the person shouting is a discredited witness or buffoon.

On the other hand, it is important to be clear about what happened. A search for evidence in relation to a real-world problem was undertaken to meet the requirements of an academic project. Sensible people do not normally change practice on the basis of a single review or study. However, belief and knowledge can be influenced by what is read and it could be that, perhaps in subtle ways, Jane's interactions with patients altered consequent to her reading. In some respects, it would be odd if this did not occur.[1] Yet because we cannot determine the comprehensiveness of her search, because the review was partial, it is feasible that located materials presented a biased picture of what was known (knowable). Given this possibility, it might be argued that changes in the way Jane interacts with patients (assuming this occurs) are illegitimate or unwarranted to the extent that (following a reading of Clifford, 2018 [1877]) the rationale for change rests on belief that was influenced by incomplete information, incomplete information can mislead, and additional (possibly corrective) information was available at little extra cost (time, resource, effort, etc.). Further, if this applies in Jane's case – when a 'good' search was conducted – the issue applies widely.

This sort of doubt or worry is easy to identify. However, it is wickedly difficult to resolve. Anyone who takes reviewing literature seriously can feel thrown when the weakness of the grounds on which conclusions rest are exposed. Once stated, these concerns sap the confidence of students and researchers. They weaken claims regards the efficiency of search strategies, and they cut away at justificatory pretensions.

Absence of agreement regards the meaning of comprehensiveness also confounds educators. In attempting to explain search processes to students, I am painfully aware that the problems discussed here remain unresolved. In a classroom setting, awkward undergraduate enquiries such as 'How many papers do I need to locate?' and 'Is my search comprehensive?' can be sidestepped by diverting attention to the assignment in hand (e.g. 'In this assignment we expect to see … etc.'). However, questions from persistent post-graduate students and researchers are more difficult to evade and, often, satisfactory answers cannot be given. Further, assessment criteria at my institution (and others I am familiar with) require that student work is graded, in part, according to whether a comprehensive range of literature has been accessed. These standards apply to first and higher degree/post-graduate work. But while I employ these mandated criteria, I do not, to repeat, understand what the descriptor refers to in a non-circular or concrete sense. When marking, I mentally substitute 'reasonable number' (i.e. local norms) and personal/subjective ideas about 'appropriate spread' for 'comprehensive range'. Yet this practice, which I am anecdotally told mirrors what others do, is manifestly unsatisfactory.

To summarise, because the phrase 'comprehensive range' lacks specificity, it is not possible to know whether this objective – whatever it means – is realised. In consequence, when all relevant literature is not located, we cannot be sure whether found sources represent the wider literature or, alternatively, whether they present a restricted and/or one-sided viewpoint. That is, while it may be possible to establish that a search is partial (by, for example, identifying relevant but missed studies), it is impossible in most cases to establish that a search is comprehensive. Further, if it is assumed that many or most searches are partial in nature, it is unlikely that comprehensiveness is generally achieved and, therefore, it may be sensible to assume that, regardless of stated intention, and in the absence of evidence to the contrary, the majority of searches only capture a snapshot of available material. This claim might seem excessively severe. Common-sense and prior learning inform interpretation, and reviewers often develop subject expertise. Nevertheless, searches are conducted to advance knowledge, understanding, thinking and learning (by, from the perspective of the standard model, answering questions). But if we cannot determine whether what is being retrieved is partial and misleading, a problem exists. Partial and possibly biased information may be and probably is influencing practice.

Systematic reviews

These problems are, in part, addressed by methodologists when they promote and emphasise the importance of approaching searches systematically.

> [L]ooking at the totality of evidence – is quietly one of the most important innovations in medicine over the past 30 years.
>
> *(Goldacre, 2011, p. xi)*

The presumption behind systematisation is that non-systematic search strategies are inadequate or irrational since knowledge, understanding, thinking and learning are not effectively or efficiently advanced by reviewing haphazardly retrieved information. And, certainly, when a review can sensibly be tackled using systematic criteria, strong knowledge claims may be established. However, regardless of whether systematisation is the best way to proceed (and I intend to object to aspects of this thing), because our grounding concepts (e.g. comprehensiveness) remain indeterminate, even systematic searchers cannot always be confident that following methodological guidance meets their objectives. They cannot, except in special circumstances (i.e. when tightly controlled keywords and phrases are summoned to address precise answerable-scientific questions using limited types of evidence), be assured that the materials they locate are anything other than a denuded assortment of what could have been found. That is, while feasible, and contra Goldacre (2011), it is not necessarily the case that well-structured systematic reviews automatically capture 'the totality of evidence'.

Systematisation takes several forms, and a distinction is often made between reviews that are conducted systematically (which, it is claimed, all reviews should be), and systematic reviews that fit or meet higher standards (Achilleas and Felmont, 2016). Systematic reviews meeting higher standards are normally performed by teams. They follow pre-agreed and pre-published methods (see e.g. Cochrane Library, 2018). They access grey and other hidden literatures, and they search out materials beyond national borders. At a minimum, both systematically conducted and systematic reviews emphasise performance and description. That is, both reviews should be rationally conducted (defendable choices are required), and sufficient detail must be provided so that others (readers) could replicate the search if necessary.

As noted, systematic reviews usually prioritise the retrieval of particular types of evidence. Specifically, research and aggregations of research (other reviews) demonstrating high generalisability will be located (i.e. randomised control trial results and syntheses of these results are sought). It is further assumed that combining this material (meta-analysis) generates results that are, potentially, more generalisable than the individual studies and reviews from which they are assembled (however, see LeLorier et al., 1997; Bluhm, 2016; Brannan et al., 2017; Edwards, 2017). Material from the apex of the hierarchy of evidence is therefore privileged, and while reviewers need to be very competent statisticians, this type of knowledge can (in principle) be learnt and comparatively agreed criteria exist for assessing success. As suggested (Chapter 3), it may be that few nurses have these skills (see also Chapter 6). Nonetheless, this approach to searching – an approach that suits particular forms of quantifiable (answerable-scientific) question – can productively inform guidelines and practice in a concrete sense, and in this way, they differ from their qualitative cousins.

Problems associated with the aggregation of qualitative research findings are discussed in Chapter 7. However, in synopsis, while qualitative reviews (systematic or otherwise) may have a great deal to offer, these reviews are less common than their quantitative brethren. They require great interpretative skill. This places heavy burdens upon reviewers, criteria for assessing success and/or competence are not agreed, they are infrequently cited by guideline writers, and their logical basis remains contested.

Relevance and research

Like other nursing students and researchers, Jane was introduced to texts that link relevance and research evidence together. This linkage has already been discussed and the pre-eminence of research as 'the' legitimate search object was emphasised in Chapter 1 by reproduced comments such as 'We were told, only reference research', and 'I tend to only reference nursing research'. The association underpins systematisation and it is also, for want of a better phrase, crudely forced in some basic primers. However, even sophisticated texts overtly elide relevance with research. For example, Parahoo (2006) asserts that "the researcher tries to identify research previously carried out on the topic' (p. 130), and Bowling (2009) states – under the subheading 'Reviewing relevant research" – that searchers will focus exclusively on research "studies" (p. 147).

This linkage is understandable. Research can provide action guiding information, and where it exists, research should be identified. The association is therefore justified when whatever question is being asked can be answered in part or whole using study findings. That said, the way we think about relevance is, I contend, at present too narrowly prescribed. Opposing current norms, even when research exists, and even when the question being addressed is amenable to resolution, it is proposed that a broader range of literatures (plural) should be considered. And, adapting Greenhalgh (2012), I suggest nurses "need to get out more, and learn from other disciplines – especially … the social sciences and humanities" (pp. 96–97) (see also White et al., 2009).

This standpoint raises its own spectrum of problems (e.g. it complicates yet again the meaning of partiality and comprehensiveness), and the vital contribution made by research to nursing is not downplayed (I would rather like to see considerably more research used in grounding practice). Nonetheless, to recap, let us suppose that Jane's search, while at least as good as others undertaken by similarly situated students/researchers, picked up just a few of the mainly research papers that might be thought relevant. And, in addition, she barely grazed the surface of accessible non-research and/or non-nursing sources. Thus, however we define relevance, her search enabled only a partial reading of the literature to take place. As noted, partial readings are perforce inadequate when whatever depth and scope of knowledge-understanding that is needed to answer or address the question or topic being investigated remains unmet. Partiality denies that an adequate or comprehensive range of sources have been accessed and, hence, the descriptor carries strong pejorative overtones. Further, since a systematically conducted search cannot sensibly aim to locate a biased and partial selection of relevant sources, partiality flouts or contradicts the goal of systematisation. This negative definition is henceforth assumed. However, it is in significant respects deeply problematic, and thinking about its problematic nature provides, perhaps, a different route through the issues so far discussed.

Partiality and judgement

The definition of partiality given above deserves careful and critical consideration. Thus, first, this definition – which was assumed in earlier discussions of comprehensiveness and representativeness – might be accused of implying that, potentially, an objectively graspable quantity of knowledge or understanding exists 'out there' that answers/addresses the purpose-question under consideration. That is, and as hinted at earlier, it could be read as supposing that if all or a comprehensive range of relevant texts were identified, a non-partial reading would be possible (relative to the question being asked or topic being addressed). Second, by absenting the searcher from what is happening, the definition ignores a key element of the search process. That is, it overlooks the fact that searches are performed by people with dynamic (unstable), normative, and emotionally charged interests.

Those seeking to locate information rarely if ever act from within states of dispassionate apatheia, and nor should they. For example, Jane chose to look at the role played by media misrepresentation of statin use because she thought some of those she cared for were adversely influenced by inaccuracies in the way information is reported and – we might infer – this troubled her. Emotion and normative values therefore played some part in attracting her to the topic, and without these subjective and personal 'drivers' the inquiry would not have been progressed. More generally, researchers are enticed to work on projects they believe are important, and individual values steer such considerations. Further, because even the most jaded and shallow of students presumably want to pass assignments, they cannot but be motivated to search for material that enables this objective (Freshwater, 2004). The myth that scientists behave in purely detached (i.e. non-emotional and non-evaluative) ways towards their objects of study was long ago dispelled by Kuhn (1970) and others (see e.g. Lyotard, 1984 [1979]; Latour and Woolgar, 1986 [1979]; Foucault, 2002 [1969]; Pradeu, 2017). However, the idea that reviewers (students and researchers) approach the literature indifferent to what, if anything, it says, continues to be perpetuated. This is wrongheaded. Location and appraisal are (regardless of systematisation) value loaded activities.

Beliefs and values in location and appraisal – a role for interests

Greenhalgh (2018) notes that people are not "empty buckets or blank slates" (p. 50) and, likewise, Hutchison and Rogers (2012) propose that the proponents of evidence-based medicine mistakenly presume that research evidence has the same impact on or meaning for whoever reads it. That is, when a report is read, readers' prior opinions and understandings are deemed irrelevant to the manner in which evidence imprints itself upon them. However, pre-established beliefs and values cannot be discounted from the interpretive process. Readers are not interchangeable or substitutable. They are not *tabula rasa* onto which research findings are inscribed. Readers have interests and concerns that influence or filter comprehension. And, since reviewers read, this line of reasoning suggests that if benefit accrues from acknowledging these prior personal commitments, searchers need to be 'placed' within the searches they perform (see Preface). In doing this, two overlapping forms of subjective response to reading can be envisaged.

First, people are motivated reasoners and they do not recognise or interpret facts in a vacuum (Kunda, 1990; Keller and Block, 1999; Rousseau and Tijoriwala, 1999; Redlawsk, 2002; Kahan, 2013; Brown et al., 2017). Hypothetically, everyone could abstractly agree that a study was well conducted (i.e. is methodologically robust). It might also be agreed that its results 'prove' a particular intervention or drug has a certain outcome (the results are universally agreed to be valid and reliable). Nonetheless, whether this study is accepted as 'evidence for' something depends on the beliefs-values and wider interests and concerns of readers. That is, a distinction can be made between externally grounded facts, and those facts being accepted as 'evidence for' something by reviewer-readers.

To illustrate the role that beliefs and values play in determining the acceptability of facts-evidence in reviews, consider the drugs Mifepristone and Misoprostol (Schreiber et al., 2018). Controversy and dispute surround their use and, colloquially, these medications have been referred to as 'abortion pills' (Adams, 2017 – see also McCullough, 2018). At present a modicum of medical oversight is required (UK law) when these tablets are prescribed. However, imagine a study that identifies a new pill which does the combined job of Mifepristone and Misoprostol but which, in addition, has no negative or unsought other effects. As research the study might be deemed flawless, and the effectiveness of the drug could be objectively agreed. Yet, this drug is designed to meet or achieve a purpose, the desirability of this objective or end goal is open to debate/contestation, defining this goal determines how our imagined study is received, and establishing goals is belief-value dependent.

Thus, reviewers who think the efficient-effective termination of unwanted pregnancy has merit will acknowledge and welcome the study. For them its existence and implications meet a "live hypothesis" (James, 1912, p. 8) or interest. And Price (1967), who explores the reasons we have for holding beliefs, suggests that assent to beliefs/propositions (here concerning the use value of the new drug) rests both on cognitive (knowledge of facts/evidence) and emotional or volitional criteria. Reviewers thus inclined should presumably recognise the existence of contrasting views and arguments (i.e. differing belief-value positions). However, reviewers with beliefs-values that allow for the termination of unwanted pregnancy can appraise the study 'objectively' – that is, they can evaluate the report *as if* personal values were irrelevant – and they may conclude that, post-appraisal, policies which make the drug available are desirable. Alternatively, reviewers who believe unwanted pregnancies should be prevented from occurring might think other methods are better suited to this goal (e.g. sexual abstinence and/or freely available contraception). Reviewers holding these belief-values may 'objectively' recognise the methodological robustness of the research report. However, they are likely to be indifferent to its findings since, from their perspective, interventions should target behaviour before fertilisation occurs. Then again, another reviewer could worry that easily available contraception encourages promiscuity. This person might again ('objectively') acknowledge the study's methodological strength but be hostile to any suggestion that the new pill be manufactured since its existence, in their eyes, promotes morally bad (licentious) behaviour. Or, 'right to life' and 'pro-life' reviewers will be antagonistic to the study. For them, the existence of the drug threatens beliefs-values about the sanctity or inviolability of life (see e.g. SPUC, 2019), and the research report in question – regardless of its methodological status/objectivity – therefore speaks to a non-issue or dead hypothesis (James, 1912).

In each case the beliefs-values of reviewers influence the way facts and evidence are interpreted. Crudely, if a reviewer's beliefs-values are socially liberal, they may recognise the study and, in addition, its findings might be situated alongside other research on the best way to move towards distribution of the drug. Socially conservative reviewers on the other hand are more likely to look for methodological errors in the study (they may be hypercritical). However, even if these cannot be found (this is an imaginary perfect piece of research), other material on, for example, post-abortion regret could be sourced and this potential might be emphasised. (In Chapter 5 epistemological theory is introduced. As will become clear, the account of the role played by beliefs and values is, in the above descriptions, coherentist.)

Second, in contrast to situations in which all reviewers agree on the methodological validity and reliability of a study, but due to pre-established beliefs-values dispute its importance (relevance and usefulness), beliefs-values can determine what constitutes evidence in a more absolute sense. For example, the American Holistic Nurses Association and North American Nursing Diagnosis Association (International) have replaced the nursing diagnosis 'Disrupted Energy Field' with 'Imbalanced Energy Field' (Larden, 2017). The website carrying this information (www.myhealingconnection.com/research) ostensibly champions evidence-based practice, and references to studies on energy fields and therapeutic touch are provided. Yet, because I do not recognise the validity of the concepts 'energy fields' and 'therapeutic touch' (as used in this context), the research listed cannot be evidence for me. I am prepared to be surprised, and while the likelihood of this happening can be bracketed with 'pigs might fly', new findings may one day emerge that confound my current beliefs-values. However, to repeat, until this day arrives, I simply deny that 'objective' evidence for these things can or does exist.

In the first example it was postulated that, although the methodological status of a study's findings might not be in doubt, the pre-established beliefs-values of reviewers could lead them to accept, ignore or reject those findings. In the second example it is suggested that reviewer beliefs-values (or in this case 'disbelief') about what counts as facts-evidence can lead to claims being accepted or rejected as evidence. Members of the American Holistic Nurses Association and North American Nursing Diagnosis Association (International) are presumably persuaded by and influenced in their beliefs by research findings. Yet, to me, this is simply hokum. Energy fields and therapeutic touch do not reference real entities and, from my position/perspective, evidence cannot exist for or verify the existence of non-existent things.[2]

Returning to Hutchison and Rogers' (2012) insight, by analogy their argument also applies to nurse reviewers and, indeed, anyone involved in EBP. No source – research or otherwise – is absorbed outside of the pre-established beliefs and values (knowledge, attitudes) of reviewers, and because of this, location and appraisal (systematic or otherwise) are informed by the interests and concerns of those conducting them. That is, the beliefs, values, and understandings of those undertaking reviews provide or give form to reasons that effect what is seen as relevant and, moreover, interests, and hence perceptions of relevance, change as new information and ideas come to light.

It is important to realise what is being said here. These claims go further than merely stating that some confluence of beliefs and values bring study topics to our attention. Instead, it is suggested that, in addition to their pathfinder potential, the beliefs, values, and understandings (often emotionally weighted) of searchers generate interests that influence the full spectrum of location and appraisal processes and, further, this influence is not being condemned. Thus, as Castañeda (2019) notes, reviews are shaped by the "interest" (p. 82) of those undertaking them and, moreover, regardless of "pretensions of objectivity, reviewers produce the fields that they avow to describe" (p. 82).[3]

Some sources are, of course, manifestly more relevant than others vis-à-vis any purpose-question (some facts cannot rationally or reasonably be denied whatever a person's beliefs-values) and, further, relevant material capable of discovery often exists in the library (loosely conceived). Thus, mindful of the critique of the definition of partiality presented above, texts can in some circumstances exist 'out there'. Indeed, for Jane, certain sources were self-evidently pertinent-relevant and this could suggest that tangibly real, identifiable and extant knowledge exists and stands apart from the purpose-questions of particular searches. This claim embodies realist assumptions (Archer, 1995), and suitably caveated it is one I have sympathy for. Nonetheless, while agreement on the texts that need to be located to meet particular purpose-questions may be found – and sometimes there is little or no ambiguity – more often than not, the idea that agreement can be reached regards some 'impartial reality' of facts-evidence is a chimera. Outside a limited and reduced range of review purpose-questions (answerable or scientific questions), either there is no agreed corpus of facts and/or when facts are agreed, their relative importance and position within wider understandings remains undecided. Searchers must therefore argue for rather than assume the relevance of whatever is included and excluded from the location process, these arguments are likely to exemplify or reflect the evaluative and normative beliefs-values of arguers, and if the necessity of interest informed argument is accepted, it follows that counter-argument and disagreement is possible. This again problematises the idea that reviewers can objectively identify all or a comprehensive range of material 'out there' because, if you think texts A, B, and C are relevant (but not others), and if I think that, in relation to the same purpose-question, texts D, E, and F are relevant (but not others), then we face a conundrum.

Elements of this problem are revisited in Chapter 5 when a 'new' search conducted into Jane's study topic is described. Nonetheless, for now, let us assume that – regards our conundrum – you and I are indeed interpreting the purpose-question and the role that particular forms of evidence play in answering that purpose-question identically. In addition, we will suppose that reasons of comparable strength and worth regarding our respective positions can be mustered. We are then left with the conclusion that each of us is defining 'all' or 'comprehensive range' differently. Maybe one of us is mistaken. Perhaps we are both wrong. However, in the absence of an external and impartial judge capable of adjudicating on our impasse there can be no final reckoning. It might be that a correct answer to the question 'what is relevant' does exist but, possibly, we do not know how to identify it. Or, as I suspect, depending on the search purpose-question, it may be that relevance cannot be stipulated without or apart from its situated context which, in this instance, includes the preestablished interests (concerns) of you and I as searchers.

Absent an external and impartial measure, we must therefore reason for rather than assume what we think is best/correct. Yet, problematically, reasoners holding radically different beliefs and values can find that their respective positions block reasoning's potential to facilitate agreement. This issue is likely to manifest itself when evaluative issues are discussed. However, it may also influence the consideration of supposedly factual matters.

Those of a philosophic bent will already have realised that an avalanche of contrasting realist, empiricist, idealist and other perspectives could at this point be invoked to explain and untangle the relationships that pertain between (to simplify) knowledge and knowers. These arguments are important, and I am very aware that the preceding discussion leaves hanging crucial questions regards objectivity and our subjective capacity to recognise and accept that which contradicts established beliefs and values. Here, however, I simply note that my proposal relates to but is different from literature appraisal methodologies that encourage searchers to detail and thereby justify, through processes of systematisation, how and why predefined search criteria were established. That is, methodologies requiring that searchers explain how and why particular types of text are accepted and rejected (i.e. the sort of detail provided in Cochrane or CDC[4] style systematic reviews). Instead, following a reading of de Winter (2016), I propose that the commitments (beliefs, understandings) and values of searchers can, if articulated, legitimately (i.e. with epistemic integrity) direct searches and reviews.

Epistemic integrity – putting reviewers into reviews

Trusted (1987) notes that: "The majority of descriptions of human activities contain explicit or implicit evaluations" (p. 17) and, moreover, many of these evaluations are moral in character. Health-related inquiries of all sorts contain or reference ethical and normative themes, and the subjective, evaluative and moral opinions of searchers are, regards these themes, always operative (Finlay, 2002b; Jacoby, 2017). Systematisation can, in highly prescribed circumstances, minimise the impact of opinion on knowledge claims. Yet to achieve this, systematic reviews collapse the form that knowledge and understanding takes by smuggling in judgements about the nature and veracity of such claims that – on reflection – we may want to reject. To give form to these abstract statements we briefly alight on the subject of justice.

While normative considerations run through much of what interests us, some topics are fundamentally evaluative. Justice is one such example. At the time of writing an unlimited CINAHL search identifies nearly 16,000 hits against the descriptor, and although CINAHL covers more than nursing, it is obvious that within this literature, nurses have and continue to demonstrate sustained curiosity in the subject. Thus, reviewers analyse sources that speak to justice (see e.g. Kayoko and Atsushi, 2014; Macleod and Nhamo-Murire, 2016; Fileborn, 2017), and they use these materials to explore and develop policy and other recommendations that directly or indirectly invoke the concept.

Reviewers are, however, likely to approach justice with preconceived ideas about what it is, requires or demands (how can they not?). These preconceptions necessarily influence notions of relevance and meaning. Yet the bulk of reviews on this topic are presented *as if* those conducting them proceeded dispassionately and objectively. Thus, although location and appraisal are influenced by the evaluative and morally charged beliefs, values and understandings of investigators, this important fact is largely ignored. These influences generally pass unstated.

Beliefs and values are troublesome when they blindly, or, to mix metaphors, rudderlessly steer literature location and appraisal. That is, difficulties are created when unarticulated and perhaps unrealised beliefs and values exert an unrecognised power over the direction and conclusions of literature searches and reviews.

> Values which one cannot identify, but merely senses implicitly, are not in one's control. One cannot tell what they depend on or require, what course of action is needed to gain and/or keep them.
>
> *(Rand, 1984a [1971], p. 210)*

Influences of this sort may be imperceptible to reviewers and, also, the readers of reviews. However, problematically, Rand (1984a [1971]) suggests that unidentified and implicit values, and we might add beliefs, cannot be defended or advanced. Moreover, while beliefs and values matter to us (indeed in some sense these things, together with our actions, are 'us'), if we are unable to establish what they entail or require, then we do not know how to sustain them. With regard to location and appraisal it is important to emphasise that beliefs and values cannot or cannot easily be extracted from interpretation. Indeed, depending upon the purpose-question being addressed, analysis and explanation may be impossible or unintelligible in their absence. However, at the very real risk of idealisation, where reviewers acknowledge and openly detail their normative positions, they can begin to control and incorporate belief-values within their work.

Note, it is not suggested that, having realised one's biases, these biases should be managed away or diluted. Rather, it is proposed that, preferably, if a reviewer can identify (and this is no easy task) that their beliefs and values bear upon the purpose-question in hand, then these beliefs and values should be recognised. This requires that beliefs-values be stated. And, potentially, this statement permits acknowledged beliefs and values to play a consistent and helpfully directive enabling role within search and review processes. Crucially, for nurses, the clarification being called for goes beyond bland statements about valuing care or compassion. Instead it necessitates a more thoughtful and exhaustive exposition, and – to repeat – accounts of this sort are not easy to do (see Preface). Nonetheless, if achievable (and this is a big 'if'), articulating searcher beliefs and values protects an important aspect of epistemic integrity. This does not mean articulation protects whatever conclusions are drawn (everyone is entitled to make mistakes). However, this type of clarification promises benefit. It might allow reviewers to understand how beliefs-values influence purpose and question setting, as well as location and appraisal more generally. And, in this way, the readers of reviews may be enabled to grasp how evaluative preconceptions (background assumptions) influenced what occurred. Thus, review readers, whose own beliefs-values similarly influence their comprehension and understanding can, once alerted, begin to form reasoned judgements about the extent to which review conclusions are affected by searcher beliefs-values.

Epistemic integrity might be likened to the sorts of declaration of interest that attach to research reports. Thus, while research into carcinogens funded by the tobacco industry may be of good as well as bad quality (funding sources can but do not necessarily influence the reliability or validity of findings), readers will clearly be concerned if the source of funding is not disclosed. In this instance lack of disclosure would, whatever the veracity of the research results, be viewed negatively. Likewise, with regard to justice, searches conducted by committed consequentialists and deontologists might seek out different evidence, and make sense of what is found in dissimilar ways. This could lead to contrasting conclusions being drawn, and the background beliefs and values of searchers are therefore of interest. Further, since the "role of the state in economic and social affairs has always been an ideologically contested issue" (George and Wilding, 1994, p. 1), when justice is linked to, for example, politics and political choice (i.e. rationing or allocation decisions), then the party affiliation or ideological persuasion of reviewers become a legitimate factor in the appraisal of those reviews.

Health and welfare policy is political all the way down (Deakin, 1994; Allsop, 1995; Klein, 1995) and, thus, when nurses concern themselves with the comparative merits of alternative methods of healthcare organisation and funding, and when justice forms a criterion in comparison, then it clearly matters if the person conducting the search favours right or left of centre policies and parties. That is, the political leaning of whoever conducts the search may influence location and appraisal, and this information should not be discounted or hidden. Indeed, regards the earlier suggestion that you might favour texts A, B, and C, while I favour D, E, and F – this situation could occur if, in conducting a literature search into the relative justice of alternative methods of healthcare financing, one of us held beliefs and values about justice that derive from or are associated with libertarian perspectives (e.g. Nozick, 1974; Rothbard, 2009), while another favoured a view of justice linked with Rawls (1971), or some version of socialism. Put bluntly, had they been nurses, Ayn Rand (1964) and Rosa Luxemburg (Hudis and Anderson, 2004) could both have performed literature reviews on some aspect of healthcare and social justice; however, their respective beliefs and values would lead them to source and interpret texts quite differently.

Alternatively – and mindful of earlier examples – where a literature search into the pros and cons of, for example, some facet of abortion is undertaken by a member of a faith community that opposes abortion on religious grounds (and assuming the searcher accepts that community's tenants), then we should expect this 'position' to be declared. Without this information, readers might unwittingly assume they are accessing an unfiltered or objective overview of knowledge whereas, actually, they are potentially reading a particular interpretation of what is known. In response it could be objected that, since every or almost every review is to some degree influenced by non-objective criteria, it is naïve or foolish to presume that a review is ever completely objective. This is reasonable. However, influence comes about by degree, and it is the degree or level of influence that readers need to be aware of. Alternatively, it might be claimed that an atheist or, indeed, a reviewer who holds no preconceived judgements about the moral or other worth of abortion should similarly declare their views – and I agree. Honesty and openness apply, if they apply at all, to everyone.

While these sorts of argument have intuitive appeal when obviously contentious topics are discussed (e.g. social justice or abortion), I maintain that the same principles apply when everyday subjects are reviewed or investigated. Thus, nurse researchers and those undertaking literature reviews into, for example, interventions designed to facilitate smoking cessation ought to make clear their opinions on smoking if or when these opinions might, or might be perceived to, influence the location and appraisal of evidence. This could simply involve stating that 'adults are free to smoke or not within the constraints of the law, and while in my professional capacity I educate patients about the risks they run by smoking, I have no wish to interfere with anyone's freedom to behave as they lawfully see fit.' Or, conversely, it may necessitate the recognition of a personal interest (e.g. 'I enjoy/dislike smoking'). Either way, these types of declaration might help researchers and reviewers to confront their own beliefs and values and, thus, they and those who consume the searches they construct – and any recommendations for practice that are made – can appreciate the significance and possibly the role of beliefs-values in the manufacture of meaning.

The point being laboured is that whenever the subject of a review has a significant normative component (and most if not all health and welfare related purpose-questions do), then – to the best of their ability – searchers should consider identifying and disclosing their preconceptions in order that the influence and impact of those preconceptions on location and appraisal can be determined. We expect to see this type of disclosure in regard to funding because, in some instances, financial sources influence the conduct and results of studies (Goldacre, 2012; Galdas, 2017) as well as clinical guideline construction (DeJong and Steinbrook, 2018; Tanne, 2018). And, correspondingly, since the beliefs and values of searchers can be similarly 'directive', these influences ought to be stated. However, this type of disclosure rarely occurs. Commonly used methodological texts dealing with literature reviews do not engage meaningfully with this topic, and nurses conducting searches are not encouraged to identify and state their normative values and background assumptions. In research, limited numbers of ethnographic studies and some of the more esoteric qualitative approaches have been interested in this issue for some time. And, as the Preface describes, researchers increasingly seek to situate themselves in their research. However, those undertaking reviews may not have thought through how their beliefs and values influence location and appraisal – and those who read the searches produced by others invariably lack (though they may sometimes guess at) this key information. Why does this situation obtain?

Scientific and non-scientific questions – revisiting relevance

Bhaskar (1997) argued that because their influence is seen as contaminatory, empiricists traditionally sought to abstract themselves from the research process. That is, it is thought that objective research is sullied when investigator beliefs and values effect experiments and/or data analysis. This approach to knowledge creation is understandable. Physics, chemistry, maths, and kindred experimental natural sciences – including a great deal of medical science – can and should seek to avoid disruptive subjective researcher influence. And, when the questions being investigated pertain to forms of 'pure' science (definitional vagaries notwithstanding), the impact of researcher beliefs-values can be limited if not eliminated (Goldacre, 2014a [2011]). However, outside of the laboratory (and sometimes within it – de Vrieze, 2017), this 'abstractive' approach to inquiry may produce impoverished conceptions of both evidence and the research process. Specifically, it has been claimed that when norms appropriate to physical science are adopted in social science and the humanities more generally, these standards engender senseless, needless, and distorting practices which, for example, speciously and impractically require that researchers be plucked from the research process (Rothbard, 2016 [1971] – see Chapter 1).

Location and appraisal are, as noted, often presented as if they are a form of research. Sometimes this association makes sense. However, traditional caricatures of science underestimate the human element in discovery and (for want of a better phrase) verification-falsification. Texts on location and appraisal snub or fly from the inevitability of subjective human influence even when unanswerable or non-scientific questions are posed (defined in Chapter 2). And we can therefore legitimately criticise unthinkingly negative attitudes towards the role and place of subjective belief-value judgement in searches and reviews when those judgements assume by default that those conducting location and appraisal ought not to influence procedures and/or findings.

That said, the evaluative preconceptions of investigators can of course overwhelm location and appraisal, and in relation to perception and perceptual justification, Siegel (2017) defines something similar to this as 'highjacking'. Kindred ideas to those of Siegel (ibid.) may be associated with cognitive penetration and/or theory-ladenness (Stokes, 2012; Cowan, 2015; Werner, 2018); and for reviewers, the danger is that unless beliefs-values are identified and subject to critique (unless a critical function is exerted), beliefs-values may derail and degrade findings or conclusions. Thus, when the beliefs and values of those performing searches and reviews engulf location and analysis, propaganda (or worse) rather than scholarship is produced. Yet, while this danger exists, we must also acknowledge that, in measure, beliefs and values are inevitably woven into our engagement with the literature and, hence, instead of pretending that these influences are not 'in play', we should recognise (through the type of disclosure described above) their impact so that searches and reviews are enhanced rather than skewed.

Recognising that normative factors run though location and appraisal problematises assumptions about relevance since, as should be clear, including or acknowledging that evaluative factors steer what is going on undermines the possibility that relevance can be defined against agreed external canons. The difference referred to here, the thing that separates what I am pointing to from standard methodologies, is that I frame the search process, and the arguments used to explain and justify that process, as fluid, iterative, and – often – normatively led. Relevance as I conceptualise it cannot, or cannot always, be neutrally established in advance of a search occurring. This alters what is meant by partiality and, hence, comprehensiveness. For, seen in this light, relevance is constructed by involved searchers before, during and sometimes after a search has concluded. This does not preclude beginning or even sticking with set search criteria and agreed agendas. Rather, it recognises that ideas and thinking about purpose-questions can develop and adjust as new information becomes available, and relevance cannot in this sense (i.e. in every situation) refer to an objectively existent 'all' or 'comprehensive range' of texts 'out there'.

Granting procedural flexibility to searchers therefore alters but in no way dissolves the problem of determining what should be included and excluded from location-appraisal. I want to allow searchers greater freedom in the sources that they utilise. And to this end, rather than being prompted to seek particular types of source (i.e. primarily research reports), searchers might be permitted and encouraged to argue for the inclusion of hitherto less exalted texts (e.g. humanities and arts 'commentaries'). As stated, the grounding assumptions operative here are that, since research maintains or occupies a largely unchallenged hegemony in the methodological literature on location and appraisal (and there is nothing wrong with research), the liberty of searchers to seek out non-research sources is abridged but, potentially, allowing a greater range of sources into reviews could have merit. Flexibility does not, however, sanction caprice. And we must refuse any suggestion that a searcher's question or topic is adequately answered or addressed by materials chosen simply by whim. That is, the elasticity being promoted does not sanction carte blanche. What is sought and what is excluded cannot solely reference personal penchant.

The problem here is that searcher preference might be judged inadequate or slanted (perhaps because the influence of searcher beliefs-values have not been thought about) by informed and reasonable others. Thus, while whoever undertakes a search ought to argue for, or be prepared to argue for, the relevance of included material, and no source should be excluded on the basis of its character alone, the final arbiter of relevance, comprehensiveness and partiality will be debate and argumentative contest rather than the voice of authoritative lone searchers (or search teams). Millsian or, possibly, Peircean threads lace through this proposal, and unashamedly rationalist and enlightenment principles regarding free speech and the value of unfettered discourse are embraced. Thus, while reasoned and rational debate do not guarantee that truth will out, their absence or curtailment is linked with truth's palliation. And, as Zeitland (1997) notes in his discussion of the *Philosophes*, discussion of the sought promoted here is "no longer merely a matter of abstract thinking. It acquired the practical function of asking critical questions … [and] Enlightenment thinking, then had a *negative-critical* as well as a positive side" (p. 2 – italicisation in original). Debate is, by this view, required to facilitate beneficial change in the world. And while the perspective advanced does not commit to any particular position regards the nature of truth, knowledge, or a knower's ability to know; it is suggested that the most defendable definitions of relevance and comprehensiveness (and by association partiality) emerge through time and in discussion between searchers (students, researchers, scholars, clinicians) and the readers, users, and benefactors of reviews.

Judgement, treatment option questions, and systematic searches

In contrast to the ideas sketched above, the standard model of searches/reviews gives, as has been stressed, significant prominence to the manner in which location is structured. For example, despite dissenting voices (see e.g. Finfgeld-Connett and Johnson, 2013), almost every published search strategy and methodological text presumes that relevance can and should be determined in advance of location (see e.g. Coughlan and Cronin, 2017; or Aveyard, 2018). This presumption, which takes 'as given' the idea that searchers are principally interested in locating research, is not without worth. And, depending upon the topic being considered, predefined inclusion and exclusion criteria may have a useful role to play. For example, randomised controlled trials and syntheses of these trials are appropriate search objects when narrowly focused treatment option questions are being addressed.

The phrase 'treatment option question' has been deployed several times already. However, what precisely does it mean? These types of question take a variety of forms. Nonetheless, the following example might be seen as representative of their ilk: 'Is dressing "A" more absorbent than dressing "B" in circumstance "C"?' This form of question is best answered using quantitative study findings, and it is not unreasonable to state that they form the bedrock of EBP and systematic review processes. However, even in the case of a simple or strictly defined treatment option question, non-research sources can augment our understanding of located research as well as the situations in which research findings are applied/applicable. And, if this is granted, it can again be suggested that greater searcher flexibility should be allowed (and in some situations, this might be necessary). After all, research results only make sense within frameworks of assumptions and conventions which – as supporting theories and normative standpoints – may be estranged or distant from the empiric findings they structure, validate and give meaning to. Background suppositions scaffold the research process, and they enfold interpretation. For instance, with regard to data use, if we include the concept of cost effectiveness in 'circumstance C', then a less absorbent dressing could reasonably and prudently be chosen in preference to a more absorbent dressing. This might occur if the difference in price between 'A' and 'B' was thought large, and the difference in absorbency was considered unimportant or acceptable. This is generally uncontentious.[5] But the point here is that these decisions involve judgement, and judgement – while ideally informed by evidence – frequently involves more than evidence.

If a literature search is conducted to aid decision making (this suggestion applies equally to research/researchers as well as practice/practitioners), and if, as in this example, that search looked only at research on absorbency – if it ignored funding, price, the realities of purchasing policy, and local clinical practice – then it would be of limited use. This does not mean it would not have value. We need to know relative absorbency rates between dressings and determining this thing is a legitimate research objective. Absorbency is partly what dressings are supposed to do or achieve. However, technical or treatment option questions are not interpreted or decided in value free circumstances and in balancing cost against treatment effectiveness, research data on absorbency provides useful but only partial information. In this instance, not much is at stake and a more thorough search could be undertaken (i.e. one factoring in price). However, it is noticeable that very few nursing research reports or reviews cost the claims for practice change they make or tacitly promote. And, more generally, the influence and remit of non-empirical (non-evidential) normative/political (evaluative) judgements in health spending and resource allocation, and the impact and role of these judgements in and on clinical decision making, is underestimated.

Which services are offered, which are cut, which drugs are purchased, and which treatments are shelved, all involve normative/political and other judgements that include considerations beyond those that research can answer. Research findings hopefully inform health related decision making. Yet knowing what 'is' cannot, without the inclusion of additional premises, tell us what 'ought' to occur. As has already been discussed, these additional premises are often provided by unarticulated beliefs and values (i.e. normatively laden background assumptions). And data are not read or used in a *wertfrei* contextual or theoretical void (Greenhalgh, 2018). If we are to grasp and critique these and other influences, if we are to comprehend our own research and clinical choices then, when undertaking a literature review, because non-research scholarship may speak to the subject of interest, we might need to examine both research and non-research sources across multiple disciplines. For example, in the case of dressing choice this might, depending on whether a narrow or broad purpose-question is addressed, involve looking at literatures associated with nursing, management theory, policy formation, and economics. Moreover, treatment option questions constitute just one of the types of problem that interest nurses, and for perhaps the majority of topics that concern us, empiric, non-empiric, scholarly, and other materials could all prove useful.

The notion that searchers must set predetermined location criteria therefore require cautious handling. The presumption is, as has hopefully been shown, problematic. It introduces ways of thinking about comprehensiveness and partiality that demand careful consideration. However, even when pre-set criteria are appropriate, default methodological preferences that prioritise research over other search objects can and sometimes should be queried. Depending upon the question or issue being addressed, the idea that research deserves preferment needs to be established rather than assumed. And this is particularly so when the topic being investigated involves significant normative or evaluative elements since descriptive empiric findings cannot substantively answer or close these sorts of inquiry. With regard to Jane's search, as should be obvious, a study that takes as its starting premise the idea that newspaper articles exert a malign influence on patient compliance is clearly evaluative to its core. To address the subject, empiric data was accessed to demonstrate the reality of this influence. Yet equally obviously, discussion of the data and recommendations for practice coupled to this discussion cannot but be heavily normative. Simply resorting to 'the research' could not, on its own, adequately inform this dimension of her work.

Further, it is feasible that whatever we access, relevance will be realised only retrospectively. That is, relevance may become apparent once we have read widely and thought carefully about what was found. This again problematises the wisdom of setting and enforcing predetermined search criteria since the possibility of following and pursing a line of reasoning through the literature in response to developing understanding is obstructed if not foreclosed by predetermination.

Alternatively, searchers could simply fail to recognise relevance. Informative sources could be identified but misinterpreted. Relevance might pass unrealised. This leads to the anodyne conclusion that what is required can be at odds with what is sought or found. Yet phrasing the matter in this way is disingenuous. As noted, the danger lies in supposing that an objectively relevant body of literature awaits the searcher who, for whatever reason, may not locate or recognise it. Instead, rather than being fixed and agreed, something designating sources 'out there', relevance may, as I contend, be more provisional. Relevance is constructed through and defended in argument. It emerges in debate and alters over time and, perhaps, this more fluid way of thinking about relevance even applies to the sort of idealised treatment option question sketched above. This line of reasoning is not new. However, it runs against the grain in nurse education and research insofar as this formulation potentially opens the door to currently marginalised sources (i.e. non-research and non-nursing material). Nevertheless, putting these issues aside for the moment, relevance and adequacy (whether all or merely a selection of sources is accessed) are in key respects context dependent.

Context and purpose

Both the context in which a search occurs and the purpose for which it is conducted are closely intertwined. However, context 'comes apart' from purpose in interesting ways. For example, searches undertaken by doctoral students are more extensive and penetrative than those conducted by first degree students, and the ability and level at which searchers operate therefore constitute contextually fluid features of location that differ from purpose (which is comparatively stable). Put another way, even where they share the same purpose, what counts as relevance and adequacy for doctoral and first-degree student searches varies, albeit that the purpose for which location takes place (establishing understandings, progressing thinking) remains outwardly the same.

On the other hand, the question or topic being investigated also forms an aspect of context. Thus, regardless of the level at which searchers operate, some location strategies can be surgically precise, narrow and swift in execution, while others are necessarily meandering, inclusive and ponderous. In this vein comparatively freewheeling non-linear search strategies have been described under headings such as 'berry picking' (Bates, 1989; Barroso et al., 2003; Booth, 2008; Finfgeld-Connett and Johnson, 2013). And because even idealised treatment option questions can involve elaborate and extravagant search strategies when the 'option' being considered is complex, the contrast drawn here differs from that made above in relation to predetermined search criteria.

Students and researchers like Jane also operate under time, resource and other environmental constraints. In many instances, these constraints prevent searchers from locating and appraising more than a smidgeon or small fraction of available sources. Constraints of this sort describe another important element of context. They oblige that limits be placed around search and review processes, and in this placement, trade-offs are made between what is achievable and what is desirable. Thus is life. However, in determining search inclusion and exclusion criteria how, rationally, is a defendable balance to be struck? How much compromise is allowable?

Problematically, constraints (e.g., not enough time) have tangible effects, and searches and reviews conducted under harshly limiting conditions generally lack value. That is, the conclusions of overly limited searches can be arbitrary, superficial, and uninformative. At worst, ill-formed reviews actively mislead. This is uncontroversial. Yet a peculiar reluctance to acknowledge this reality is observable and, for example, textbooks and other teaching resources display an odd coyness when they insist that all or a comprehensive range of relevant sources be located, but – definitional problems notwithstanding – do not concede this is infrequently accomplished or possible.

Constraints of this sort also encourage students and researchers, often with educator or supervisor connivance, to fall back on or invoke situational justifications to excuse inadequate location and appraisal practices. Thus, 'Yes', searches are performed in limiting environments and searchers, often through no fault of their own, undertake work that is poorly supported and under resourced (Paley, 2016). However, 'No', recognising that problems infest the conditions searchers operate within does not vindicate or validate their outputs. It may be that scraps of knowledge, incomplete understandings, and underdeveloped thought gained through drastically limited searches, offer marginal improvements upon even-more limited knowledge, even-more restricted understandings, and even-more restricted thinking; that is, the condition existing before a limited search was performed (though how this would be established remains unclear). Nonetheless, even though a search may achieve the best that can be realised in constrained circumstances, where too partial a range of sources is located – and, hence, a search's conclusions do not reflect what is known/knowable, key understandings are not identified, and/or interesting and informative ideas are not grasped – then, because that search does not meet the purpose it was undertaken to achieve (i.e. non-trivial learning), it should, as rubbish, be unceremoniously binned.

Excuse and compromise

Phrases such as 'overly limited' and 'too partial a range' are circular or tautologous since they already presume that which they seek to reveal. Nevertheless, stating that rubbish should be discarded starkly and deliberately articulates a provocatively hard line. This is not a position that everyone will accept. However, by presenting the issue in this way I here emphasise the challenge to 'attitudes of excuse' and the retreat to apology ('this is all I could achieve, so it will do') that, together with a reformulation of the concept of relevance, are important elements of this book.

That said, the difficulty of what is being proposed cannot be evaded. Genuine and sincere attempts to get to grips with the literature place arduous demands upon researchers, who may be aware they are only scratching the surface of topics, as well as clinicians, who seek knowledge and understanding so that they can act in the world. Further, when we contemplate what must be determined before knowledge/belief sufficient for action can legitimately be claimed, standards regarding evidence and/or reasons for accepting knowledge/belief quickly spiral upwards, and at higher levels, scepticism is encountered (Horgan, 2016).

Sceptics recognise that knowledge/belief always rests on shakier or less secure grounds than we suppose or would like and, in consequence, it is naïve to assume that even the broadest definition of relevance (including one assuming that all information could be accessed), can protect knowledge/belief in any final sense. This is important. The challenge posed by scepticism is profound and its anarchic or destabilising influence is not often given due prominence (Pritchard, 2019). That said, while the suspension of judgement or *epoché* called for by sceptics in the face of uncertainty (see e.g. Perin, 2010) may be an appropriate response in some circumstances, we normally avoid insecurity about knowledge/belief claims by implicitly utilising less stringent parameters for truth justification which, I here assume, comes about by degree. That is, in logic and psychology, justificatory reasons for holding knowledge/belief claims are cumulative. Confidence in the reasons we have for knowledge/belief thus build or amass incrementally. Justificatory warrant is rarely simply present or absent, and regards searching for and reviewing literature, while more rather than less evidence and information is generally desirable, this viewpoint allows us to break with the idea that all relevant literature must be sourced. This objective, as previously and repeatedly stated, is practically unobtainable in most if not every instance, and again as noted, the proposition might speciously be taken to imply that if all or even a comprehensive range of literature was sourced (assuming the meaning of these phrases could be established), key facets of scepticism would be vanquished. Neither proposition holds and, thus, although determining relevance and establishing when enough material has been located is, in relation to a search's purpose, clearly difficult, judgement, and a willingness to articulate and defend choices made is a vital part of explication.

Let us grant then that knowledge and understanding does not need to defeat radical scepticism (which is impossible), it merely has to be good enough for the purpose in hand. The term 'good enough' is, of course, question begging. Nonetheless, positively, the phrase brings to the fore the place and role of thoughtful deliberation while, negatively, the requirement places heavy burdens on deliberators. I therefore acknowledge and have no wish to underestimate the problems that students and researchers face and, crucially, I do not think ideal or perfect searches or reviews are, bar exceptional circumstances, possible. Nevertheless, if we accept that knowledge, understanding and thought generally remain 'unfinished', and the 'open' concept of relevance introduced earlier allows and embraces the idea that, in important respects, location and appraisal cannot be closed, then the idea that contextual constraints can justify limited searches and reviews lacks credence. Tensions obviously exist between reading widely to gain the best understanding possible, and reading instrumentally to inform decision making amid the clattering urgency of clinical practice. 'Good enough', which differs from the concept 'reasonable' (described earlier), offers a compromise between extremes. However, the point stressed here is that arguments deliberately favouring the acceptability of reduced knowledge, understanding and thinking are unsustainable (Parkhurst, 2017), and if nurses honestly intend to benefit patients, then knowingly engaging in poor practice is unacceptable.

Notes

1 Originally published in 1877, William K Clifford's 'The Duty of Inquiry' (part of *The Ethics of Belief*) states that: "No real belief, however trifling and fragmentary it may seem, is ever truly insignificant; it prepares us to receive more of its like, confirms those which resembled it before, and weakens others; and so gradually it lays a stealthy train in our inmost thoughts, which may someday explode into overt action, and leave its stamp upon our character for ever" (2018, p. 3). In Chapter 5 it is suggested that 'old' texts can have value for reviewers. Further, it is proposed that methodologists may be in error when they direct reviewers to ignore dated sources. Although the argument is yet to

be made, Clifford is exactly the type of scholar whose work still merits consideration. Thus, while *The Ethics of Belief* does not present research findings; nonetheless, anyone interested in "questions at the intersection of epistemology, ethics, philosophy of mind, and psychology" (Chignell, 2018) would do well to consult this interesting and influential resource. Indeed, if the thrust of Clifford's (2018 [1877]) argument is correct, where reviewer interests focus on such questions, they will be at fault if they do not do so.

2　It might be protested that, for example, racism is 'real' (has real effects) albeit that what racists postulate (their notion of race) is unreal. This is not, however, the existing/non-existing dichotomy referenced here.

3　An objection here might adopt something like Camus' (2013) insight that "Logic founded on passions reverses the traditional sequence of reasoning and places the conclusion before the premises" (p. 17). That is, reasoning which is overly influenced by passion/emotion begins rather than ends with a conclusion. This danger is acknowledged. However, as Camus (2013) ably describes, in the absence of values (themselves in part informed by emotion), reason can have only arbitrary or temporary endpoints. Reason becomes skittish.

4　Centers for Disease Control and Prevention – www.cdc.gov/

5　Or, rather, it is mostly uncontentious. Complications can, however, easily be envisaged. Professional codes of nursing conduct/ethics assert, for example, that nurses should follow 'best practice' and give 'best care' – yet – when the meaning of these phrases is not clarified, muddle easily results. Thus, the UK NMC (2018) state that effective practice involves acting "in line with the best available evidence" (section 6), and it is therefore arguable whether 'second' or even 'third' best treatments/interventions (e.g. less absorbent dressings) can permissibly be used (i.e. used when absorbency is the stated rationale for dressing application/choice). Alternatively, section 2.2 of this document asserts that nurses must "empower people to share in decisions about their treatment and care". 'Sharing', like evidence can be variously interpreted. Nonetheless, including patients in decision making allows that 'they' along with 'us' might have a role in choice taking and, perhaps, patients could prefer the 'best' (most absorbent) dressing irrespective of cost. That is, 'they' may choose the option that best meets their interests, and we cannot assume that patients will adopt 'our' assumptions regards cost-benefit trade-offs or indeed treatment goals. This issue deserves greater attention. The literature on EBP tends to assume harmony rather than discord in clinician-patient interaction. However, Greenhalgh (2018), who notes the reality and importance of clinician-patient power imbalances, points towards potential tensions.

5

NURSING AND NON-NURSING SOURCES

An ordinary search (part III)

- A new search is conducted.
- Theories of epistemic justification are introduced.
- Research and scholarship are contrasted.
- Non-research scholarship can be a relevant source.
- Context and purpose are revisited.

Specialist health related websites and databases were employed by Jane to locate research. In addition, guidelines and policies concerned with statin use were accessed, and the history of guideline and policy development was investigated. Further, contradictory and contrarian medical opinion on the subject was sought, and studies dealing with media distortion and statins were found. Compared with other work produced by students/early career researches, this was, to repeat yet again, a good search. However, simultaneously, it was also a decidedly partial search and this once more drags us back to the question: how deep and how wide should reading (location and appraisal) go?

Things overlooked

Typifying the weakness inherent in predetermining search criteria, as her study progressed, Jane became aware that aspects of the topic she was investigating were not covered by or discussed in the sources located. Failure to find what we seek often follows the implementation of poor or less than satisfactory search strategies. However, it may be that, as I have argued, standard approaches to searching are sometimes inadequate, and if this possibility is granted, we should consider what is omitted from ordinary search protocols. Specifically, what potentially informative sources are overlooked by the methods we employ?

Nursing interests frequently transgress or cross disciplinary boundaries. That is, the questions and topics that interest 'us' can also be of interest to 'others', and in such instances, alternative (complementary and/or contradictory) non-nursing literatures exist on 'our' subjects. Since these non-nursing literatures can inform (support and/or challenge) understanding, and since we want to access or develop the best understandings possible, it can be difficult to determine where a search should begin, go, or end.

In Jane's case, while a small number of demonstrative tabloid newspaper and magazine articles were accessed to highlight the sort of misreporting that patients are exposed to, a more vigorous exploration of non-nursing and non-health related materials might have been charted. As a nurse, Jane sought to understand how misinformation influences the beliefs and behaviours of patients in order that she could, forearmed, challenge misconceptions and provide better care. However, given her aims, and mindful of the importance of the topic, although approaching the search from a nursing and/or health-based perspective made sense, it also meant that non-nursing and non-health resources were effectively discounted. Academic media repositories, for example, were not scrutinised even though these collate more information about the nature and extent of media influence than nursing and health related sites do and, likewise, literatures on communication of the kind held in dedicated psychology and social science databases were overlooked. Exploring these repositories and databases would have unearthed information and ideas with direct clinical applicability and, thus, although standard search methods can, depending upon the purpose-question being addressed be 'sensible', they may also be restrictive and obstructive when, by channelling the focus of a search too tightly, pertinent other material is missed.

Wide reading is, despite comments in Chapter 1, supposedly prized. And throughout higher education, students are exhorted to evince extensive reading in submitted work. The number and breadth of papers that need to be accessed and incorporated into written assignments for wide reading to be demonstrated normally remains wisely unspecified. However, in an extensively shared and generously praised piece on research essays and literature reviews, Rosenberg (2017) suggests that five to six references are appropriate for a 1,500-word essay, seven to eight are typical for a 2,000-word essay, a 4,000-word essay should have between 15 to 16 references, and a 6,000-word essay 18 to 25 references. Moreover, at the time of writing, internal documents at my own institution suggest that between ten and 15 references are an appropriate number of sources for a 3,000-word undergraduate assignment, and these figures are not dramatically out of kilter with Rosenberg's (2017).

The absurd and frustrating illogic built into these types of statement have already been noted. Suggestions of this sort pay no heed to the nature of the purpose-question or issue addressed. They are formulaic, stifling, and idiotic (just in case I am at all unclear, I don't like them). Nonetheless, beyond numbers, wide reading is clearly not a problem free activity and, for example, where a topic is best explored by considering (in part or whole) non-nursing sources, and when non-research as well as research texts are considered to be legitimate search objects, how, given that we may not be familiar with their location or comprehend the background theories they assume, are non-nursing research and non-research literatures to be sourced and understood? Can non-research literature legitimately influence practice when that practice is supposedly evidence based? In summary, how are we to access and make sense of the sorts of texts that do not get picked up by searches conforming to standard model precepts when those overlooked works promise to contribute something of note to whatever purpose-question we are concerned with?

A.n.other search

Aware of these questions, and having become interested in the subject of Jane's investigation, I conducted a quick search of my own. This identified numerous 'hits' that Jane had overlooked and, indeed, depending upon the search terms that are used, many hundreds of highly pertinent texts are potentially identifiable. These include nursing *and* non-nursing but explicitly health-related resources such as Bazian's (2016) NHS 'Behind the Headlines' post *Heart attacks linked to media statin reports,* Nabi and Prestin's (2016) report into the influence of sensationalistic news stories on health behaviour motivation (published in *Health Communication*), Kriegbaum, Liisberg and Wallach-Kildemoes' (2017) cross-disciplinary work on statin use and media coverage (*Patient Preference and Adherence*), Demasi's (2018) critical narrative review of what she describes as the 'Statin wars' (*British Journal of Sports Medicine*), and Nordestgaard's (2018) commentary on 'why' the media are negative about statins (*European Heart Journal*). In addition, my search threw up material that, while applicable, was more tangentially aligned to health. See, for example, Shen, Sheer and Li's (2015) meta-analysis into the impact of narratives on persuasion in health communication (*Journal of Advertising*). And it located decidedly non-health related but I would argue germane texts like Feinstein's (2015) position paper on education, communication and science in the public sphere (*Journal of Research in Science Teaching*).

Depending on how Jane's purpose-question is interpreted (see Chapter 3), every one of these resources contains information and ideas that could have contributed to her study, and while Nabi and Prestin's (2016) report is the only source cited (above) that is available through CINAHL – in relation to her work – a strong case could be made for the assertion that each was relevant. That is, each source might productively have informed the object of her study, this informing would have advanced knowledge-understanding-thinking (learning) and, therefore, each could have legitimately been included/cited.

I also ordered a book that I had long meant to look at, namely, Adolf Guggenbühl-Craig's *Power in the Helping Professions* (1971, German edition; 2015, English translation). This work critiques, from a Jungian psychoanalytic perspective, how the commanding position and expert knowledge held by analysts, social workers, teachers, doctors, nurses and other 'helpers' configures, sometimes negatively, professional-client relationships. I know little about psychoanalysis. Nonetheless, to the extent that health education attempts to produce behavioural change in patients/clients through the provision of professionally approved and evidenced advice, and since the communicative strategies this entails can, from the perspective of patients/clients, be simultaneously both supportive and disempowering, the theme of Guggenbühl-Craig's book – a thoughtful examination of the witting and unwitting misuse of power by professionals, and the often unconscious resistance offered by those experiencing help to what they interpret as helper domination – appeared to overlap with aspects of Jane's study.

This correspondence was confirmed when, in conversation, Jane suggested patients occasionally preference media reports over expert instruction to, in part, repel or block the paternalistic overtones that healthcare educators are perceived to exhibit (note, clearly this is a synopsis of what was said – no one actually talks in this way). And if this insight is correct, if her comments contained an element of truth, then nurses ought, when discussing media misinformation with patients, to be mindful of the power and status inequalities that infuse nurse-patient interactions and, also, the danger of imagined or actual professional overbearance accompanying this imbalance. On the face of it, Guggenbühl-Craig's (2015) book therefore looked as if it could scaffold arguments in her work, and while only one explicit reference to nursing is made in the text (p. 125 of the 2015 Spring Publications edition), the book offers a novel and insightful account of key aspects of communication. Thus, had I been undertaking her study, I would have referenced the book.

We might then conclude that no problem exists. I should simply have introduced the work to Jane, and if it met her needs, she could cite it. End of story. However, before rushing on we ought to consider the following points.

Like the majority of 'new' materials noted above, Guggenbühl-Craig's (2015) book would not be located using recommended or taught search strategies and, for example, while my university identifies several hundred hits for Guggenbühl-Craig in non-health related library databases, CINAHL records no results against his name (at the time of searching). The work is therefore effectively invisible to nurses like Jane who follow taught review protocols, and while alternative and imaginative approaches to systematising search stratagems have been suggested (see e.g. Ayala, 2018), these are rarely promoted. Moreover, I cannot now remember when or where I initially heard about the book and, problematically, while contingency and luck play a role in most if not all activity, searches conducted by students and researchers should not rest on serendipity or impulse. Some logical defence must presumably be offered or available that explains and rationalises the presence of identified material, and 'just knowing' about the existence of an included source – i.e. Guggenbühl-Craig – undercuts the systematisation that the standard model requires to be evidenced.

Foundationalism, coherentism, and reliabilism – epistemic justification

The issue here is that, as a journal reviewer and educator, I am pushed to assess and grade literature searches using performative rather than outcome measures. Thus, searches conducted systematically are prized above those which are unsystematic. This does not mean that only systematic reviews have worth (Thorne, 2018b). It does mean systematisation (a systematic approach) should be demonstrated by searchers. Standard descriptions of systematisation clearly state what good practice involves (e.g. predetermining inclusion-exclusion criteria, prioritising the location of research etc.). Yet the value judgements contained in such practices (e.g., slighting by implication non-research), mostly pass unnoticed. Alternatively, focusing on performance (was a systematic approach to searching described?), overlooks the outcomes obtained (was informative and interesting material found?) and, arguably, this places the proverbial cart in front of the proverbial horse since, perhaps, what matters is what we find rather than how we find.

To make sense of what is going on, epistemic theory is introduced. Foundationalism, coherentism and reliabilism reference categories of theory which explore ideas concerning epistemic or knowledge justification. That is, theories about how or on what grounds we know the things we think we know – assuming we do indeed know them. (For extended discussion on this subject see Griffiths, 1967; Shatz, 1983; Sher, 2016; Long, 2018.)

Foundationalists, for example, hold that basic non-inferentially justified beliefs support or ground inferentially derived beliefs. This sentence is somewhat difficult to comprehend. However, it summarises an epistemological approach that addresses or takes seriously the problem of infinite regress that arises if we presume every belief invokes or makes use of other beliefs that, in turn, rely on other beliefs *ad infinitum*. Foundationalists escape this regress by asserting that some beliefs do not require justification. That is, some beliefs do not need to be justified or defended. They simply are true/correct.

Coherentists, on the other hand, reject foundationalist concerns with inference. They discount inference's attendant problems and, instead, they suppose beliefs ought to be understood and assessed in relation to wider belief systems. What matters to a coherentist is that belief systems are coherent, and to be coherent, systems need to demonstrate consistency, cohesiveness and comprehensiveness (and these are all, clearly, tricky words). Coherentists, we might suppose, would concentrate on what is located in a search and, in particular, the relationship of ideas across texts, rather than how something is located.

Alternatively, reliabilist theories of knowledge/belief justification have become increasingly popular in recent decades. These theories propose that truth conduciveness rests on the reliability of belief forming processes underpinning knowledge/belief. How a belief is formed is, from this perspective, crucial in deciding whether that belief is justified (i.e. can be justifiably held). And it might be proposed that, in key respects, insofar as systematisation 'stands in' for reliable belief forming processes, the heavy emphasis given to systematising search procedures embodies analogous reliabilist insights.[1]

Linking epistemic justificatory theories to search and review procedures stretches their respective (disputed) definitions. This must be noted. Nonetheless, these ideas can be recruited to 'explain' key components of the standard model of reviews. Thus, the valorisation of systematically structured searches makes use of what look like reliabilist procedural criteria to justify or underpin claims regarding the truth conduciveness of conclusions and, moreover, the validity and reliability of research report findings rest or are determined by reviewers on essentially reliabilist grounds. Coherentist reasoning on the other hand comes into play when results are brought together in or for evaluation. That is, arguably, while procedural reliabilist assumptions inform both location processes and the assessment of individual research reports, coherentist principles are deployed in the later stages of assessment. Coherentists are interested in whether or to what extent ideas and/or facts cohere or can be synthesised with other knowledge/beliefs. Further, though to a lesser extent, it might be wondered whether earlier discussion regards comprehensiveness and partiality echo coherentist tropes.

What then of Guggenbühl-Craig's (2015) book? As stated, this would not be identified using standard model review strategies, and the manner of its location and its subsequent presence amidst search results cannot then be explained or justified against reliabilist assumptions (of the simplified variety described here). The text therefore occupies or falls into something of a liminal space or no man's land. The manner in which the book was identified and retrieved are inexplicable against systematising criteria, and while we might not want to reject or lose what Guggenbühl-Craig says (on coherentist grounds he aids understanding), how this understanding can be 'slotted into' review processes remains unclear. Indeed, from the perspective of an adherent to standard model strictures, the text is awkward to incorporate or cite.

This issue differs from but falls within the same arena of problems to those identified in Chapter 1 when inclusion-exclusion criteria were chastised for failing, in practice, to do the thing they are supposed to do. That is, in most instances inclusion and exclusion criteria can be variously interpreted and (excepting Cochrane or CDC style reviews) it is often difficult – it is frequently impossible – to ascertain why particular texts are used or rejected. In both instances, when lax and/or overly precise inclusion-exclusion parameters are set, and when apparently germane texts such as Guggenbühl-Craig's are 'found' outside of systematising search structures, reviewers – and review readers – who wittingly or unwittingly preference reliabilist 'type' assumptions concerning epistemic credibility can encounter or run into logical conundrums in describing and/or comprehending the comprehensiveness, partiality and relevance of search results.

Research and scholarship are not synonymous

While *Power in the Helping Professions* is a relatively short scholarly monograph, it is nonetheless considerably longer than most research reports. The work therefore takes more time to read and make sense of and, as stated, hard pressed students and researchers may not enjoy the luxury of being able to engage with these sorts of extended text. Yet, what is thereby lost?

Although some of the questions that nurse reviewers ask can be adequately addressed using short research papers, we also pose questions and develop interests that demand engagement with extended texts that may or may not be research reports. However, if taught search methods and the cultural or normative expectations that accompany them encourage nurses to locate and read only brief texts, if it is presumed that short research reports are all that need be accessed, then the knowledge and wisdom contained in longer and/or non-research texts cannot make themselves known. As an educator I am, moreover, prompted and sometimes obliged to recommend and use only electronically available texts (e-texts), and this potentially aggravates further problems associated with 'short' reading. Positively, since library stocks can be denuded, the use of e-resources should ensure that all recommendations are available to all networked readers at all times. But, negatively, access to e-resources is far from universal (Farahnaz, Azadi and Azadi, 2017), not every book and paper has been digitised, and gaps in digitisation most readily apply to longer and dated works.

Pre- and post-registration (licensure) primers on the subject of search and review often, as previously noted, recommend that any text which is more than a few years old should not be sourced. Cronin, Ryan and Coughlan (2008), for example, recommend that a "maximum timeframe" (p. 40) of between five and ten years be set. Neill (2017) suggests five. The rationale for this is self-evident and reasonable. We do not want outdated research findings influencing nursing practice. However, as soon as we allow that non-scientific and sometimes scientific questions can make use of and therefore validly 'look to' non-research texts, the importance of age limitations evaporate. Further, dated is not the same as outdated. To be outdated implies, in this context, that new and better (i.e. more accurate or more sophisticated) interpretations have become available. In contrast, being dated purely refers to age and this condition, in itself, does not necessarily mean that improved understandings exist. The idea that research and non-research texts have, merely by dint of age, nothing to say or contribute to contemporary practice is thus logically indefensible, and unless old ideas have been falsified or superseded, they should not be discarded. Similarly, assumptions that presume the irrelevance of non-research scholarly texts must be defied. Neither supposition is secure. Both wither upon reflection.

Therefore, when students and researchers investigate topics that are explored in long text form, but only short texts are accessed, then, difficulty notwithstanding, we need to reconsider the implications and acceptability of such practices. In addition, when relevant topics are discussed in older research and non-research works and when, despite the passage of time, the content of these texts still resonate with our interests, we ought to rethink ideas around both the form in which texts are accessed and the span of years searches cover.

The thrust and direction of these arguments are not, however, universally accepted. And it should be noted that Guggenbühl-Craig's (2015) book, written at the end of the third quarter of the twentieth century, is exactly the type of text that standard taught search strategies seek to avoid. Thus, not only is the work old, it is also not research (as traditionally defined). And although the work sympathetically unpacks a topic that, within the context of

Jane's study, might be considered relevant, the conclusions or themes it describes are not action guiding. Or, if that statement is too strong, the propositions and opinions it offers are not action guiding in the same way that evidence supplied by a well-conducted randomised controlled trial is supposedly action guiding. Arguably, this criticism could also be levelled at non-generalizable qualitative studies and reviews of those studies (Thorne, 2016b). Yet, this aside, Guggenbühl-Craig does not offer instruction. The book does not report experimentally deduced facts. It does not 'tell' nurses what to do. Therefore, since professionals read to inform practice, and since this text cannot inform practice in any straightforward sense, its usefulness is open to dispute.

Those who would deny the book a place in nurse searches and reviews include senior colleagues (educators and researchers) with whom I work. For these people, since the metrics used to reward achievement in UK University Nursing Faculties/Departments overwhelmingly prioritise research, non-research outputs inevitably lack worth. Research is therefore valorised, and scholarship is marginalised. This allows scholarship to be conceptually 'folded into' research, and scholarship and research thereby come to be treated as essentially interchangeable terms. My colleagues do, grudgingly, grant non-research scholarship an independent but heavily prescribed role in nurse writing. That is, scholarship is seen as useful when it can be recast as theory that researchers thereafter investigate. And in keeping with this perspective, Aveyard, Payne and Preston (2016) allow reviewers to search for "theoretical literature … to provide a framework for your empirical review" (p. x). However, this outlook presents a curiously circumscribed vision of intellectual accomplishment and the value of that accomplishment, and it is one I reject.

If pushed, I suspect those who are reluctant to grant non-research scholarship a firmer base in nurse searches and reviews hold, almost certainly unwittingly, to two positions. First, they probably prefer forms of ideational presentation that lean towards or might be associated with analytic rather than continental philosophy or ways of thinking. Distinctions between these schools should not be overdrawn and these descriptors reference loose and disputed 'attitudes' rather than clearly defined objects. Nonetheless, in broad brush terms, analytic writing values focus, succinctness, clarity of exposition, and reasoned argument – whereas continental philosophy and writing is, by comparison, more expressivist, evaluative and emotive in form. Nurse writing displays a great deal of fondness for evaluative writing. Yet, while we must acknowledge the simplified caricatures that constitute the preceding generalisations; Kanterian (2015) notes that, applied to knowledge claims, short research papers often trump wide ranging scholarly monographs and commentaries for those of an analytic temperament and, I suggest, my colleagues evidence this disposition in their diminution of long-form scholarship.

Second, those with whom I disagree may accept a sharp distinction between epistemic discovery and justification. It has thus been argued that while ideas can be discovered or come from anywhere – including scholarly writing – only scientific methods and practices can justify or warrant claims about the world (Bluhm, 2017). This binary categorisation has a long history. It is commonly linked to positivism and, in particular, Carnap's *The Logical Structure of the World* (2003 [1928]), albeit that both earlier and later emanations of the bifurcation exist (Hoyningen-Huene, 1987). Intellectually the discovery-justification dichotomy is intriguing. However, it is too severe. It shrinks what counts as evidence by giving too much weight to particular accounts of science, and while scholarship is a constituent element of research, it also exists and takes place apart from research. It is the value of this 'apartness' that needs to be asserted.

If theory and scholarship are simply and only instruments that provide stepping stones to empirical investigation, then the possibility that theory and scholarship might exemplify, stimulate or contribute to understanding in their own right is refused. This emasculates the worth and role of theory and scholarship and, regrettably, my associates take up this enfeebling position when, by allowing research a domineering role, they all but merge research with scholarship. However, although non-research scholarship can and sometimes does further immediate instrumental or professional needs, it does not always do so and the worth of, for example, *Power in the Helping Professions* (Guggenbühl-Craig, 2015), derives both from the ideas it contains and the critical stimulus it provides. Potentially at least, scholarship of this sort enables other knowledge to be situated or placed within wider perspectives of thought and comprehension (*à la* coherentism), it challenges existing ways of thinking, and it upends taken for granted assumptions. Intellectual writing and scholarship therefore has value regardless of science's ability to licence what is said; and as Lynch (2012) persuasively argues, non-research texts can contribute to doxastic (belief) systems through the generation of ideas "some of which are true in virtue of corresponding to the facts but others of which – such as our philosophical and ethical beliefs – are true simply by being part of the explanation" (p. 134). Crucially, scholarship and the humanities/arts, broadly conceived, may provide "real reasons" (ibid., p. 135) for conviction, albeit that they do so in ways and on grounds that differ from those provided by objective, public, replicable, science.

Interpreting non-research scholarship

If we permit that non-research scholarly texts can sometimes be legitimate sources of information and ideas – and hence constitute acceptable search targets – how should these sources be interpreted? Aveyard, Payne and Preston (2016) acknowledge in a single sentence reference to books and book chapters that "theories and concepts … may be related to your work" (p. 84). However, the manner in which meaning is attributed to or derived from non-research scholarly work remains obscure.

I later critique the ability of nurses to meaningfully understand and apply research report findings (Chapters 6 and 7). Nevertheless, tools, frameworks and benchmarks exist that purportedly assist in assessing the method and methodological strength of research reports. Thus, if research is conducted robustly, if quantitative measurement techniques are valid and reliable, and/or if enough information is supplied regarding data collection and evaluation in qualitative work then, all other things being equal, we might grant that results and findings, while fallible and contingent, provisionally stand. (I am definitely not arguing that nurses should not read research.) However, against what metrics are we to gauge Guggenbühl-Craig's (2015) scholarly acumen? To what extent does and should the stature of the author vouchsafe the claims being offered? Is the book's internal logic and power of argument the thing being assessed? Or is its persuasiveness, its impact on the reader, the decisive factor? And if, hypothetically, you and I both read the book and I say 'this is fascinating' and you say 'this leaves me cold', what then?

In one sense, if we allow that interests and beliefs-values influence understanding and receptivity (discussed Chapter 4), then differences in responses to sources are to be expected; there may be no 'problem' to explain. That said, readers can presume greater liberties in identifying the aspects of scholarship that are valued and found useful than are generally taken with research findings. That is, while the accuracy of and meaning attaching to report findings can be and often is fiercely disputed, disagreement is anticipated and expected when interpreting scholarly work. A common feature of this disagreement involves the evaluation of scholarly argument[2] and, for example, confronted by your cold indifference, I could respond by proposing that, albeit from radically divergent positions, since other noted scholars' advance kindred observations to those made by Guggenbühl-Craig (2015), his ideas may be worth listening to. Thus, for me, a semblance of similarity or crossover exists between Guggenbühl-Craig's (2015) observations and passages in, amongst other works, Nietzsche's *On the Genealogy of Morals* (2013), Plato's *Republic* (2007), Rand's *Atlas Shrugged* (1996) and Smith's *Theory of Moral Sentiments* (2010). These texts vary enormously. They include theoretically informed and polemical fiction as well as political and ethical philosophy. And without difficulty any number of sociological and psychological (including the aforementioned position paper by Feinstein, 2015) or policy and political papers (see e.g. King, Schneer and White, 2017) could be added to this list. Nonetheless, the point pressed here is that these texts might be recruited to sustain Guggenbühl-Craig's (2015) main proposition or focus as I comprehend it, and an argument can be constructed with a view to altering your indifference.

To be carried, detailed explanations of these claims are required. Moreover, I am not proposing that we vote on truth. Piling up supportive sources (here, listing those making kindred points) carries little weight. And while (the Thomas theorem) "If men define situations as real, they are real in their consequences" (Merton, 1948; 1995), simply asserting a position rarely makes it so. Nonetheless, that said, to some extent Guggenbühl-Craig's (2015) exploration of the misuse of power by mostly well-intentioned authoritative helpers, and the defensive reactive responses generated among those being helped, finds echoes in the work of other scholars, and by analogy (mindful of coherentist principles), presumed consensus lends credence to his comments.

In riposte, you might counter that arguments from resemblance may, in actuality, be based on illusory connections (perhaps the result of representativeness heuristic/bias). Or, even when justified and hence defendable, resemblance, used to substantiate claims for the importance of works of non-research, differs markedly – as noted – from claims to importance grounded on methodological criteria of the sort associated with experimental research. Another way of presenting this issue is to recognise that, although understandings inferred from non-research scholarly texts, as well as artistic products (including fiction), can augment, embolden, and give form to our thinking, the stimulation and ideas provided by these sources differ in kind from knowledge delivered by empiric research. Again, it would be wrong to overemphasise the dissimilarity referenced. Nevertheless, while abstract reflection and reproducible scientific facts both influence thinking/belief, they do so on the basis of contrasting rationales.

In determining relevance, you could (and probably should) also challenge my ability to appreciate or comprehend work written from a Jungian perspective. That is, how confident can I be that I realise what is being said when the ideas I think I grasp are built upon and incorporate theoretical concepts that are unknown or unfamiliar to me? Moreover, while psychoanalytic claims have been extensively disputed (Murray, 2018), even if accepted, this approach to understanding is variously interpreted and not all interpretations are (presumably) of equal merit. How then can readers who lack a developed knowledge of Jungian psychoanalysis and its use or application judge the value of such texts? Problems around understanding apply widely and, for example, while difficulties associated with reading non-research scholarly works are highlighted here, similar issues infest research report interpretation.

Thus, clearly, research reports often reference esoteric methodological, epistemological and (sometimes) ontological theories – and issues concerned with interpretation and understanding surface when these studies are read. As Chapter 1 records, comments such as 'How much of this paper do I need to understand?' and 'I don't do statistics. I don't understand them. I don't read them', point towards the sorts of difficulty and insecurity that many students experience. In her study, Jane identified quantitative research papers that incorporated dense statistical analysis. However, neither she nor I are trained to interpret this material and we might then ask, when reviewers cannot comprehend how study findings are derived from statistical tests, can they sensibly accept and act on those findings? I presume not. Alternatively, the majority of qualitative research papers identified by her search asserted rather than demonstrated that particular themes emerged from the analysis of interview transcripts. Yet if we must accept claims (here emergent themes) before they are taken up and assimilated as knowledge/belief, and if acceptance requires that the derivation of findings (themes) be meaningfully rather than trivially understood, then insofar as the processes underlying emergence remains shrouded from readers, this again suggests findings should not be accepted or acted on. That is, qualitative emergent themes cannot be granted the status of knowledge/belief. (These arguments might be situated within reliabilist frames.) Issues of 'interpretation' therefore crop up in relation to research and non-research products alike, and the problem of interpretation represents or is yet another underexplored topic within methodological texts.

Language

Regards Jane's search, as can be seen, sticky issues are readily pulled out from what was a well conducted but otherwise standard investigation, and these questions in no way conclude those that could be asked. For example, although research and scholarship relevant to nursing takes place in the non-English speaking world, except for a few highly resourced reviews, this literature is largely ignored by those who, like me, lack the linguistic skills necessary to access it.

Guggenbühl-Craig is not a nurse. Nonetheless, we can use his work to make a general point and ask, what was the status of *Power in the Helping Professions* (2015) before it was translated into English? It obviously existed. However, the insights it contained were only accessible to German speakers. English is the lingua franca of scientific discourse, and research papers published in English accumulate more citations than their non-English brethren (di Bitetti and Ferreras, 2017). Huge amounts of potentially informative non-English research and scholarly work nonetheless exists albeit that the overwhelming majority of this remains untranslated. Moreover, just as I could not read Guggenbühl-Craig's work before translation, non-English speaking nurses are unlikely to benefit from scientific and scholarly discourse written in English. This problem is further exacerbated for nurses working in impoverished and poorly resourced regions, and while, no doubt, poverty generates more pressing worries – we will not hear their voices, and they cannot hear ours.

Researchers are aware of problems associated with removing non-English speakers (and those who lack fluency) from studies performed in countries where English is the primary language spoken (Frayne et al., 1996; Kurt et al., 2017; Bernier et al., 2018; Smith et al., 2018; Staples et al., 2018), and the publication bias this generates is recognised (Scherer et al., 2018). However, when it comes to reviews, although the issue is acknowledged (Cochrane, 2017; Rasmussen and Montgomery, 2018; Polo et al., 2019), nurses regularly exclude non-English studies (see e.g. Butun and Hemingway, 2018; Northwood et al., 2018), and little attention or emphasis is given to locating and appraising non-English texts. Reviews performed by nurses thus tend to overlook the impact of reduced cultural and linguistic diversity in accessed sources. The influence of this lacuna on comprehensiveness and generalisability passes unremarked and, arguably, lack of interest in this topic signals or might be described as a significant blind spot.

Context and purpose revisited

Following discussion, Jane decided that she would not cite Guggenbühl-Craig (2015). She agreed that it spoke cogently and directly to elements of her study. It also dealt with themes that went unaddressed in the papers her search located. However, Jane guessed, probably correctly, that no credit would accrue from embarking on a discussion of the book or the subjects it covered in her work (a study prepared in part completion of a higher degree). She recognised that the text would in all likelihood be unknown to those reading her work and, moreover, given the constrained and constraining nature of marking criteria, supporting an argument with unusual sources (i.e. ones requiring extended explanation) might conceivably count against her. Yet this endpoint is deeply disturbing.

Guggenbühl-Craig (2015) was introduced to draw out some of the issues that get over-looked when the standard model of reviews is applied unthinkingly. It is thus perfectly reasonable to ignore this particular text. However, it seems intuitively wrong that interesting and possibly significant lines of inquiry are shelved because nurse educators and journal reviewers find, or are perceived to find, it difficult to accommodate unusual material and topics. Derisory comments such as 'I tell them, go to CINAHL, one or two official sites – Oh – and the Code. That's it' (Chapter 1), should have no place in a university setting, and anyone who voices such sentiments ought to feel and be ashamed. Students, researchers, educators and clinicians need to obtain the best understandings possible, and where best understanding is obtained from wide and careful reading, including reading that steps outside of traditional nursing sources, then that is what ought to happen and be encouraged.

As stated, location and appraisal are undertaken for a purpose and within a context. The purpose is, broadly speaking, to map a body of knowledge, to identify key understandings, and to stimulate thinking (learning). More narrowly, while specific purpose-questions may best be addressed by locating and appraising research, it is also feasible that non-research sources should in some circumstances be consulted. In the preceding pages I have suggested that non-research scholarly works can contribute to knowledge, understanding and thinking in some if not all instances and, where this is the case, these texts need to be classed as relevant sources (i.e. legitimate search targets) in the same way that research is classified. By outlining my case in this way, I may have inadvertently given the impression that wide reading is, within reviews, only 'about' non-research texts. I certainly want to open up the range of sources that nurses deem valid search objects, and I intend to situate this opening up within an argument favouring interdisciplinary discussion and debate about the nature of relevance. However, my aim is inclusionary rather than exclusionary. I would like to add sources to those seen as acceptable. I do not want or mean to suggest that research reports are invalid sources of information (that would be foolish). Thus, appropriate material – both research and non-research – can, depending on the purpose-question being considered, be found in nursing and non-nursing literatures. That this needs to be stated is somewhat peculiar. However, almost every nursing guide on the subject of literature searches and reviews focuses overwhelmingly on the location and appraisal of research and, moreover, students and researchers are frequently pushed to prioritise nursing sources.

With regard to the contexts in which searches take place, students and researchers attempt, among much else, to convince assessors and journal reviewers that systematic and rigorous procedures have been followed. That is, procedures appropriate to the level of study being progressed or the research project being performed, a manner commensurate or attainable within prevailing constraints. Nonetheless, these caveats disclose or hint at the 'rub' which exists between purpose and context.

Mapping a body of knowledge and identifying key understandings are rarely if ever achieved absolutely, and thinking clearly has no end point. Yet it would be strange to state that the purpose of location and appraisal was to establish 'a smattering' of knowledge, 'a chance selection' of understandings, or 'a quota' of thought. We may never entirely meet the purpose-question for which these activities are undertaken. However, while the goals reviewers seek to attain are unashamedly ambitious, context, on the other hand, curtails aspiration. Contextually, location and appraisal are relatively situated. Thus, while doctoral students are expected to know and have addressed the writings of major academics and theorists pertinent to their field of study, it would clearly be inappropriate and unfair to hold first-degree students to the same stringent criteria. Further, neophyte students and early career researchers are not chastised for failing to achieve excellence (almost always an impossibility). Nevertheless, although we have to respect and acknowledge the reasonable adjustments that context demands, too much reasonableness offers a backdoor to pragmatic constraints ('not enough time'), and if these sorts of consideration go unchallenged, if they assume or are allowed too great an influence ('therefore what is done is sufficient'), searches and reviews will fail the purpose they are supposed to accomplish. They might never achieve 'good enough' let alone 'best' understandings.

Excuse cannot then be permitted to justify or rationalise overly guarded approaches to engagement with the literature. Contextual constraints are real, they have concrete effects, and these embedded realities may be difficult to shift. Further, clinicians should and must prioritise immediate care needs over other requirements. Nonetheless, when conducting reviews, if nurses acquiesce or act in what Sartre termed 'bad faith' (1996), if we accept without question or critical challenge 'attitudes of excuse' – that is, if we apathetically assent to wretchedly limited goals even when we are aware that alternative and possibly more enlightened ways of working exist – then students and researchers, indeed all of us, will fail to locate and make sense of apposite and informative sources and, hence, the searches and reviews we perform cannot but be unduly fractional and dispiritingly inadequate. Frankly, allowing the constraints we operate within to overwhelm or dominate the context in which location and appraisal take place compromises the purpose these activities seek to meet.

Cumulatively, too easy recourse to attitudes of excuse – or simply excuses – contributes to nursing failing to develop a language capable of describing the activities it engages in. Or, where narrow reading prevents us accessing useful knowledge, understandings, and insights; we may fail to develop defendable ways of articulating and talking about those activities. Should this occur, nursing will not be able to grasp the issues it faces, and to the extent that this inability hampers problem identification and resolution, clinical practice will suffer. These statements do not sustain the Sapir-Whorf hypothesis or support any of its abundant idealist offspring (Deutscher, 2005). That is, they do not sustain the idea that language's structure determines perception and the categorisation of experience. They merely state something less contentious. Namely, when excuse permits denuded searches to be accepted and acceptable, nurses will not articulate as well as they otherwise might the problems they confront, and this must damage or harm patient care.

Notes

1 To hopefully make what can be complicated ideas accessible, the epistemic justificatory theories introduced here (and mentioned earlier) are presented in simplified form. A great deal of nuance is thus omitted. Each theoretical category can be further differentiated. Alternative or intermediate positions exist, and every theory is open to challenge. For example, in contrast to the idea that it is a separate and/or isolated principle, Goldberg (2012) suggests process reliabilism is a version of foundationalism, and a vindication of coherentism. Reliabilists are, moreover, confronted with the problem of defining reliable belief forming tokens or processes (Swinburne, 2001). And Klein (2005; 2012), who identifies with infinitism (a perspective that embraces the regress worrying foundationalists), notes that where equally coherent but competing belief sets exist, coherentists must choose between belief sets. This makes coherentism look a lot like foundationalism since, while the advocates of each position must decide where they stand, their reasons for choosing can lack depth/grounding. That is, ultimately, foundationalists must assert that 'such and such' is a foundational belief and, likewise, coherentists are required – confronted by equally coherent but opposed belief sets – to pronounce upon or claim a favoured option in the absence of external or objective criteria. Haack (2014) makes a similar point albeit using different arguments.
2 Where a purely subjective or personal insight is gained from reading non-research material, and when this insight does not sanction or produce action in the world, external or public justification for that insight is not required. However, I here presume that where insight informs action in the world, explanation and/or justification is potentially necessary.

6

REVIEWING QUANTITATIVE RESEARCH

- Nurses are not educated (enabled) to interpret the statistical tests that quantitative researchers use.
- Reviewers who cannot interpret and read statistical tests do not meaningfully understand how findings are derived.
- If nurse reviewers cannot determine how findings are derived, they should not presumably accept or use those findings to inform practice or research.
- Difficulties of comprehension are heightened when 'big data' and other complex forms of quantitative study are encountered.
- Nursing's understandable interest in values (e.g. 'being caring') may inadvertently exacerbate problems associated with statistical competence.

Review methodologists' lavish attention on research papers. Yet lack of preparedness or ability on the part of many (not all) nurses, and professional reluctance to learn from and work with other disciplines, handicaps key elements of research appraisal. Methodological innovations in fields external to nursing exacerbate or highlight these difficulties insofar as advances in non-nursing domains bear upon and implicitly challenge the way nurses conduct searches and reviews. (While we tend our walled garden, outside the world is in flux.) To illustrate just a few of these developments, this chapter examines issues thrown up by 'big data', while Chapter 7 – which focuses on qualitative research – discusses 'active citation'.

What is not happening

In Chapters 6 and 7, we outline the problems that hamper the analysis of located material and weaken or detract from the quality and value of reviews performed by nurses. However, to begin with, it is important to be clear about what is *not* happening. First, a tremendous amount is written about quantitative and qualitative critique. Most of this material is useful, and anyone who accesses published sources should make some sense of whatever it is they are reading. Thus, nurse reviewers can and do successfully evaluate research papers, and it is merely proposed (albeit vigorously) that facets of appraisal require additional consideration. Second, at no point is it suggested that research is unimportant. Research findings productively and appropriately inform nurse thinking and it would be good to see this happening even more than it does at present. Indeed, had I a magic wand, the nursing curriculum would allocate considerable additional time to the study of research methodologies-methods, statistics, and the integration of findings into practice. Moreover, nursing actions (care) ought to be grounded on or consider research evidence whenever this exists and, frequently, this is precisely what happens. Large numbers of nurses surmount the difficulties outlined in the next two chapters, and when problems are not overcome, individuals continue to do the best that they can to interpret and appraise study findings.

Thus, reviewers often produce outstanding work, and where snags occur no blame attaches to nurses for not being able to do things they have not been educated or enabled to do. I am not, to repeat, anti-research – and while strong arguments can be mounted in favour of opening up the range of sources that nurses access and, also, increasing cross- and interdisciplinary engagement; favouring a version of EBP, and broadening out the diversity of material considered in reviews are not incommensurable objectives. These goals need not be opposed.

Methods and statistics

Moule (2018) recognises that many nurses "find the results and analysis section of a research article difficult to understand" (p. 129). Nonetheless, research reports are important in reviews, and appraisal aims to establish whether study findings are warranted. To determine warrant or trustworthiness, reviewers need to assess reports at a depth or level commensurate with assessment allowing an informed judgement to be made about the value of the object being appraised. This crudely boils down to the question – should these results be trusted? And when, for whatever reason this is not possible, when the warrant or trustworthiness of findings cannot be vouched safe, the results or knowledge claimed in the study being reviewed ought not – unless other 'good reason' exists – to inform practice/research.[1]

To establish warrant, reviewers need to know whether correct methods were used, and methodological texts aimed at nurses sensibly devote considerable space to explaining research methods. Much less attention is, however, given to statistics. Distinguishing between methods and statistics is a tad peculiar given that, in quantitative studies, research methods and statistical tests are closely intertwined. Thus, methods employed in data collection influence which statistical tests can be used and, also, statistical tests designate the method by which data is analysed. That said, it is noticeable that while reviewers are directed to examine the mechanics of study design (e.g. the manner in which subjects were recruited, the validity and reliability of measurement tools, the presence or absence of randomisation, forms of blinding, etc.), little and sometimes no attention is given to unpacking statistical and data analysis.

> An important component of critical appraisal is evaluating the statistical analyses used in the research report…. [However] The analysis of statistical methods, results, and interpretation is the most challenging part of critical appraisal for two reasons. First, many clinicians are inadequately prepared for the task…. Second, the quality of reporting statistical results in many reports is inadequate to support clinical decision making.
>
> *(Mays and Melnyk, 2009, p. 125)*

Rather than commenting on appraisal in relation to all methods, this chapter focuses on statistics. And, bar the most basic of surveys/designs, it is suggested that quantitative researchers often employ tests that are not introduced or explained in under- and post-graduate nurse education (Mays and Melnyk, 2009). The statistical tests which are used may be understandable 'in principle', and were a statistics course to be successfully completed, reviewers could comprehend some if not all of the tests deployed in quantitative studies (assuming adequate reporting practices). However, in the absence of training, many and perhaps a majority of the statistical devices encountered in quantitative papers will not be meaningfully understood by nurse reviewers.

> [Y]ou [the reviewer] will need to become familiar with the characteristics of the main types of study type to be included. For example, if you are planning a review of ran-domised controlled trials you will need to be able to recognise the key features of such a study, their likely limitations, and the consequent threats to validity that they may pose.
>
> *(Booth, Papaioannou and Sutton, 2012, p. 45)*

Booth, Papaioannou and Sutton (2012) arguably direct reviewers to consider statistics since their use represents a key feature or 'characteristic' of, in this case, randomised trials. And, self-evidently, if tests are not chosen or conducted appropriately the credibility of findings collapse. Yet in their otherwise excellent book, little attention is given to statistical analysis. Generalisation and statistical significance are discussed. However, these topics are covered in comparatively brief notes, and statistical tests are not substantively engaged. This is important. More might have been said.[2]

Reviewers who take up questions capable of empiric resolution (Chapter 2's answerable questions) frequently locate quantitative reports. Quantitative evaluation generates any number of conundrums. However, the need to make sense of the tests that produce findings is rarely headlined. Meaningful appraisal involves evaluating statistics *and* methods more generally. Yet, since statistical understanding is largely underplayed in the methodological texts nurses access, threats to the validity of study findings may go unnoticed. It is therefore sensible to ask – what do reviewers need to comprehend about the statistical tests that appear in the studies they appraise?

The first of two views – *my position*

In my opinion reviewers need to grasp both that the correct statistical tests were chosen, and that those tests were properly used (i.e. run). These, to me, are vital parts of quantitative appraisal. Moreover, establishing that tests were suitably run involves, I suggest, under-standing actual calculations. Absent this understanding, reviewers do not comprehend how findings are derived in anything other than a trivial or inconsequential sense.

Developing earlier claims, crucially, if reviewers cannot determine how findings have been derived (when they are unable to meet the criteria set out above), without other 'good reason', warrant has not been established, and unwarranted findings should not be recognised or utilised. Put another way, accepting and using results without understanding and having confidence in, amongst other things, the (reliabilist) statistical processes that produced them means findings are classed as evidence (and may therefore influence practice/research) on the basis of guesswork, hope, fiat or assertion and this, I contend, is the very antithesis of critical appraisal and EBP (Lipscomb 2014b; 2016b).

Conversely, a significant tension exists within my position and this needs to be acknowledged. Thus, although statistical tests are often difficult to understand, it is proposed that, as stated, meaningful appraisal requires that they be understood so that the warrant or trustworthiness of research results can be recognised. Yet, simultaneously, large and complex tests – for example, those incorporated in what are here termed 'big data' studies – may outstrip the ability of even experts to comprehend or realise how they work/function. This, if correct, appears to suggest that in relation to 'my position', the findings of big data studies cannot be assessed (their warrant remains indeterminate) and, hence, these results cannot be accepted. That is, they cannot legitimately inform practice or research. This is clearly daft. Scale and complexity cannot be allowed to 'rule out' study findings, and a means of reconciling this tension is therefore required.

Moreover, although 'authority' and 'evidence' need not be antagonistic, EBP has been positioned in opposition to authority-based practice (Gambrill, 2018 [1999]; Gifford et al, 2018). And absent an established and defendable evidence base, in certain circumstances, actions are sensibly and reasonably undertaken on the basis of authority (command) alone. If this is granted, perhaps the results and interpretation of statistical tests can likewise be accepted on authority? Maybe reviewers can safely presume that the right test was chosen and has been used or run appropriately when, for example, the report in which it appears is placed in a respectable peer reviewed journal (i.e. a journal with an authoritative reputation)? If true this would defeat my position. However, as will be shown, the presumption does not hold.

Authority and belief

In clinical practice, if Professor Consultant Samantha orders that patient Jones be subject to intervention 'x' it would be foolish for Nurse Smith to refuse to comply simply because she is unaware of the rationale supporting the instruction. It is reasonable, absent evidence to the contrary (and 'evidence' can be stretched here to include subjective experience), to obey expert or authoritative commands/instruction, particularly if the intervention is deemed urgent. And while we might and probably should ask questions and seek to understand why we do what we do (and Professor Consultant Samantha ought to be prepared and able to explain her reasoning), complying with authority claims is valid in many if not every instance. In addition, adapting Moore (2017), at the level of clinical practice we do and perhaps should accept the authority of expert institutions (e.g. NICE,[3] Cochrane, or the CDC) when the cost of checking what they recommend, or the complexity involved, outstrips our ability.

By analogy, in everyday life it is probably sensible to accept that manmade or anthropogenic climate change is happening, and that state sponsored childhood vaccination is beneficial (on aggregate), even when we are aware of heated controversy (alternative positions), but have not personally investigated and assessed evidence regarding these issues. Indeed, it may be that even very able individuals cannot comprehensively evaluate and confirm the warrant and trustworthiness of evidence around complex subjects (here climate change and childhood vaccination). Possibly, either so much evidence exists that it cannot all be reviewed or, alternatively, interpreting evidence might demand so many skills that no one person – however, well equipped and trained – could complete the task. Additionally, as Moore (2017) ruefully notes, climate change and vaccination deniers may be well informed about evidence on these topics, more informed at any rate than most of those who decry denier positions.

Permitting authority a legitimate role in decision making complicates but does not wound my position. Moore's (2017) insight, for example, can be linked to previous comments (Chapter 4) regards the role of values in belief formation. That is, scientific conclusions are not value free constructions (Hicks, 2014), their reception or rejection is values dependent, and when considering claims based on authority, values clearly play a part in how these are received. Thus, evidence from the US suggests Liberals and Democrats are more likely to believe in and be concerned about manmade climate change than Conservatives and Republicans, and this left-right divide is also discernible in Europe (McCright, Dunlap and Marquart-Pyatt, 2016). Indeed, the influence that political and other value dispositions (e.g. those linked to religious orientation, social class, etc.) have on climate change acceptance is now well established (Hornsey et al., 2016; Stanley, Wilson and Milfont, 2017). And political, religious, class and other influences (including race, and parental beliefs regards immune functioning) differentiate vaccine deniers, refusers, sceptics, and acceptors (Freimuth et al., 2017; Ward et al, 2017; Krok-Schoen et al., 2018). Values, to state the obvious, influence belief.

Where values reference issues with 'political' content (i.e. many health-related topics), disagreement should be expected and, for example, clinicians encounter problems discussing health with patients when health is negatively impacted by environmental factors carrying climate change implications (Alame, 2018). Yet, in addition, beliefs are also (by degree) rational or irrational. Hansson (2017) dismisses the concerns of climate change and vaccination deniers by suggesting their views are based on irrational pseudoscience, and Gorman and Gorman (2016) likewise recognise the significance of irrationalism in such debates. Irrationalism, in these instances, is associated with denier values. However, while I believe deniers are mistaken, stressing the influence of values in belief formation runs – we should note – both ways. That is, my willingness to 'rationally' accept science-based arguments I have not personally investigated on authority (i.e. on the authority of those who appear to legitimately 'speak for' scientific methods and practices) is as much a product of the values I hold as rejection of these arguments/authority (and the embrace of irrationality) is the product of denier values. Moreover, there is I suspect a tendency for writers to highlight the way values influence the reasoning of those they disagree with, but not themselves. That is, since 'we' are obviously rational and right, those we disagree with must be irrational, emotionally labile and normatively biased.

Note, it is not suggested that because all viewpoints are (by degree) evaluative, all positions are in some sense equal. Nurses making exceptionalist claims are criticised later in this chapter (see also Preface), and exceptionalism encourages or allows irrationalism. Good arguments can be mustered to support the proposition that some positions are irrational and mistaken. Nonetheless, even those who are rational and right in the positions they adopt do not accept or conceptualise those positions in value-free ways, and this requires acknowledgement.

Allowing that it is rational to accept claims based on authority does not, in addition, mean those claims are correct. Regardless of the role that values play in disposing us to accept or reject authority claims, when performing or reading a review, it remains the case that EBP and the purpose of critical appraisal more generally runs counter to a thoughtless submission to authority. Claims made by authoritative people and bodies are, in this context, provisional and their influence is circumscribed. This must be stressed. Authoritative institutions such as the World Bank have made serious errors in understanding systematic reviews (Haddaway, Land and Macura, 2017), and medical experts regularly make catastrophic mistakes. For example, not only did Kohn, Corrigan and Donaldson's (1999) Institute of Medicine study *To Err Is Human* estimate that medical errors in US hospitals result in anywhere between 44,000 and 98,000 unnecessary deaths per year – but:

> Even when using the lower estimate, deaths due to medical errors exceed the number attributable to the 8th-leading cause of death. More people die in a given year as a result of medical errors than from motor vehicle accidents (43,458), breast cancer (42,297), or AIDS (16,516).
>
> *(Kohn, Corrigan and Donaldson, 1999, p. 1)*

Recent approximations suggest earlier work significantly underestimated deaths from error. Makary and Daniel (2016) situate medical error as the third leading cause of death in the US (see also Giardina et al., 2018), and while precise figures are difficult to come by (Shojania and Dixon-Woods, 2016), healthcare workers – whether working as clinicians or reviewers – must question authority whenever they suspect decisions are mistaken. What then is legitimate authority? And, two related questions – when is it sensible to do/not do as requested, and when should research findings or guideline or review recommendations/results be accepted/rejected?

It has been suggested that authoritative figures (e.g. Professor Consultant Samantha) should be prepared to explain and thereby justify orders and, in a similar vein, we might note that authoritative guidelines (e.g. those produced by NICE or the CDC) are not 'abstractly' authoritative. Rather, just as the soundness of the research process is judged against procedural or broadly reliabilist criteria (Chapter 5), so the commanding status of authoritative guidelines rest on the confidence users have in the processes employed in their manufacture. This confidence comes from published descriptions of what and why guidelines writers did as they did, and this information enables readers to refer back to and check the evidence and reasoning upon which claims are grounded. This detail provides a rationale for belief (acceptance) and in principle, should users wish to consult, confirm and/or challenge guidelines directing their actions, they can do so (and finding 'fault' in these sorts of document is regularly done by nurses taking higher degrees).

Thus, while we do and frequently must act on the basis of authority, valid or 'acceptable' authority allows and facilitates (in this context) the checking of reasons and reasoning. In clinical settings it is generally sensible to meet the authoritative demands of expert seniors. However, when assessing evidence, reviewers need to unpack the claims they are considering. When quantitative studies are being examined, assessment requires that the detail of statistical tests (including calculations) be understood and, as will be argued (below), peer review is an inadequate basis on which to judge statistical warrant. Reviewers cannot simply accept quantitative results because they appear in authoritatively respected sources (e.g. 'trusted' journals).

The second of two views – was the best test applied?

My position, outlined above, emphasises the importance of reviewers engaging with 'actual calculations'. However, mine is not a popular position.

> [I]t is important that you understand what the results of a study mean, rather than have a detailed understanding of the statistics used in the studies.
>
> *(Aveyard, 2018, p. 60)*

Aveyard (2018), for example, proposes that reviewers can adequately determine what a study's findings mean without understanding the statistical tests used to establish those findings. Alternatively, Janet Barker (2013) states that:

> all you really need to know is what is the best test to apply in given circumstances, what it does and what might affect its validity/appropriateness. It is not necessary to understand the actual calculations involved.
>
> *(Barker, 2013, p. 89)*

Barker does not think it necessary that reviewers understand actual calculations, and following extended discussion with colleagues, hers appears to be the majority opinion on this topic among nurse educators (or, at least, those known to me). Nonetheless, Barker's statement (made in regard to critical appraisal in EBP) still imposes a substantial burden on appraisers, and to understand what is involved even in this reduced conception, I here interpret Barker as committing reviewers to a four-stage process. This description fills out or goes beyond Barker's actual statement. Yet, hopefully, I do not misrepresent what she meant or intended. The picture I put forward of what might and possibly should occur is idealised. In many senses it is absurd. However, the following comments are, I believe, logically assumed in Baker's claim.

Barker (2013) wants reviewers to establish that the "best test" (p. 89) was applied. This supposes that a single best test is available (agreed upon) in all instances and, perhaps, this assumption is less secure than we imagine (Gelman, 2018). Nonetheless, the premise can be accepted insofar as, if a 'less than best' or inappropriate test was used, results might not tell us what we want to know and/or they would be less informative than they could be. Indeed, if the wrong test is used the worth and significance of a study's findings presumably evaporates. Caveats aside, establishing that the best test was employed is therefore a basic or grounding aspiration for quantitative reviewers. How then might this be achieved?

First, reviewers must understand the test or tests that were chosen. This is clearly pivotal. For the moment I park what understanding involves. However, in this context understanding is not a binary object. It is not simply present or absent but, instead, develops or is present in degree (we normally have more or less rather than total or no understanding). There must then be a point at which 'sufficient' rather than 'full' understanding is achieved. Yet nursing methodologists do not discuss when 'enough' understanding is held or how one might know this thing is achieved. Further, when confronted by a lack of knowledge (or insufficient knowledge), there is more to understanding than simply 'looking something up'. This issue is discussed shortly. Nonetheless, if a reviewer comes across an unknown test they can seek guidance, and it should be possible to appreciate or learn something about the test employed. That said, significantly, even if reviewers establish that an appropriate test was chosen, this does not in itself answer the question 'was the best test used?' Appropriate and best are or can be different things. Thus, a test might be appropriate without necessarily being best (but not vice versa).

To determine 'bestness' we need to know about alternative tests that could have been but were not chosen. Therefore, second, contender tests that were available but not used should be identified. Contender here references similar tests. That is, tests that might have been substituted for those used had, possibly, minor changes to method protocols or research aims been made (examples are given below). Contenders may not exist. However, this needs to be determined rather than assumed.

Third, mindful of the range of actual (chosen) and contender tests (if available), reviewers should employ a measure to compare and judge between tests. Thus, reviewers need to evaluate the appropriateness of tests used against overlooked/unused alternatives, and in this way (through comparison) what was best can be devised. Comparison can involve considering whether tweaks to methods/aims might allow more powerful and hence possibly better tests to be employed.

Finally, fourth, having employed measures to establish that the best test was picked (and assuming it was), reviewers must decide that tests were suitably rather than unsuitably run, and to this end (putting to one side 'actual calculations'), factors or variables affecting validity and/or appropriateness within the circumstance of each unique study require determination.

A crucial aspect of my interpretation of Barker's (2013) statement, the thing I want to emphasise, is that to establish the best or most appropriate test, appraisers need to compare tests used against potential contenders that were not used. (Parallels between this claim and those lodged in Chapter 3 regards alternative purpose-question wordings are easily drawn.) For this to occur reviewers must possess or have access to extensive statistical knowledge/literacy, and a nuanced acquaintance with methods and the interplay between methods, unique circumstances, and tests also appears necessary. This level of statistical ability and method/methodological insight is not, however, widely held. And what is proposed rarely happens. (To repeat, I appreciate idealisation is involved here.) Yet if these steps are not implied by Barker's statement, if – for example – the element of comparison is removed, how are reviewers to establish that the best test was chosen? In what other way is best being determined? Can reviewers settle this fundamental feature of quantitative research without following something like the procedure outlined here? Or is establishing mere appropriateness (a significantly lesser claim) sufficient?

That said, if the idea of comparison is taken seriously, if to identify the best test we need to compare and contrast used tests against possible alternatives, reviewer difficulties balloon. Explicitly, where similar or comparable tests to the ones employed exist, we must acknowledge that identification is, in anything other than very simple cases, rarely straightforward. For example, two by two contingency tables with low counts can be analysed using Fisher's exact test *or* chi-square. Fisher's gives a precise P value, whereas chi-square (which is easier to use) provides only an approximate P value. All other things being equal – and they rarely are – researchers should presumably pick Fisher over chi-square (though whether the extra effort involved is worthwhile is difficult to judge). Alternatively, while, strictly speaking, z-tests and t-tests are distinguished in use according to whether observation data are independently taken from a normal distribution with an unknown mean and known or unknown variance – when large sample sizes are considered, both tests can, sometimes, be considered interchangeable (a consequence of central limit theorem). For both of these examples, researcher preference, and the objectives and logic of a study legitimately determine test choices. However, where differences obtain between kindred and similar tests, while it should be possible to identify better and therefore best tests against specified criteria, excepting professional statisticians, few nurses are educated to make these sorts of decision (I certainly am not).

As is obvious, even if something like the four-step process outlined here makes sense, its implementation would encounter significant difficulties. Maybe then, we should try to find another way through the problem. For example, some tests are more popular than others (Zellner et al., 2007), and recognising this, Barker (2013) outlines commonly encountered forms of descriptive and inferential test. She thus explains that descriptive statistics employ or talk to means, frequency distributions, percentages etc., while inferential statistics include *t*-tests, correlations and, for example, chi-squared tests. Perhaps then, rather than assuming that nurse reviewers can and should identify and compare tests in the manner described above, it would be better just to educate reviewers (students and researchers) to comprehend regularly encountered tests? We might wonder whether agreement could be found regards which 'common' tests should be taught. Nonetheless, this suggestion is voiced by colleagues with whom I work and, practically, most of us are only aware of or familiar with tests we frequently use or assess.

Focusing on commonly used tests would make sense if reviewers only appraised work containing such tests. However, large numbers of tests are referred to in published work. The complexity and sophistication evidenced by these tests often outstrips the introductory descriptive-inferential outlines found in nursing texts (even progressive ones like Barker's). And unless reviewers restrict themselves to assessing papers that only employ tests they are familiar with (which would be peculiarly limiting), they cannot but encounter tests they do not know and, in some fashion, these need to be understood.

Contra the idea that reviewers only need knowledge of commonly deployed tests, to identify that the best test was used, it seems reviewers must have or seek out theoretical knowledge about every test they encounter. In addition, since both usual and unusual tests can have similar and possibly interchangeable analogues, reviewers appear to require considerable understanding. But this is ridiculous. Reviewers do not and cannot know about every test (no one does), and confronted by a new or unfamiliar test, guides (e.g. text books and educational internet resources) will, as noted above, be accessed. True – but – this assumes reviewers can interpret and make sense of the information contained in guides, and we might want to pause here.

Significant percentages of nurses lack ability and confidence in mathematical and statistical use (Warburton et al., 2010; Barker, 2013; Hart and Little, 2017). Yet if establishing that the best test was chosen requires that reviewers possess epistemically meaningful rather than scrappy or superficial knowledge, and if evaluation involves comparing and judging chosen tests against competitors, reviewers need a developed overview of the field of available tests. This requires considerable learning and, perhaps, continued and ongoing immersion in the statistical literature (at which point the nurse reviewer might better be thought of as a statistician). Confronted by the unfamiliar, guides will be sought. However, meaningful understanding can be difficult to glean in this way. I here assume that understanding involves more than simply determining that 'this' test does 'this' thing and – *good* – that is what the research under review did. Moreover, a great deal of prior knowledge is required to interpret guides which, in regards to statistics, may make assumptions of readers that readers cannot meet. Therefore, suggesting reviewer's reference guides to find out about statistical tests they are unfamiliar with is both sensible *and* questionable.

Further, when we think about what comparison entails, the prospect and difficulty of measurement hoves into view. Thus, 'best' assumes comparison and comparison involves measurement. It is only in relation to stated measures (criteria) that we can say 'this' test outperforms 'that' test. Or, 'this' test is superior to 'that' test 'because'. For example, if one of the criteria for determining bestness is having a precise P value, then – if appropriate – Fisher's exact test should be chosen over chi-square. However, if ease of use is a criterion (and I suspect it rarely should be), the reverse is true. (I here set aside questions about P value 'worth'.) In addition, arguably, in some circumstances, it might be that reviewers ought to either think through or actually run tests (using published data) to establish what works against defined measures. New skill sets would be required for this purpose, and these skills are not currently taught outside specialist statistical courses. However, to repeat, unless statistical tests are compared in some way, we cannot determine which is best/better. Comparison is meaningless – it does not occur – without some form of measurement. And if a measure is used, presumably this involves running data through tests and evaluating which best meets the measure? Or, if this does not happen, what does it mean to say that a test is best for a given purpose? Without comparison and measurement 'best' is a meaningless term.

Finally, Barker (2013) stresses that tests are used "in certain circumstances" (p. 89), and deciding within the context of each unique study the factors or variables that might affect validity and appropriateness in a wider sense – i.e. in certain circumstances – is no easy task. Numerous considerations bear upon statistical choices, and assessing their relative influence plays a role in comparing and judging between alternative contender tests. Yet advanced statistical and methods acumen (as well as experience) is required to determine this thing, and the moment we try to articulate what this involves in a substantive sense, outlandish and overbearing burdens are heaped upon reviewers.

I must therefore be wrong regards the four-step process outlined above. Published reviews do not take the steps which, I believe, are implicit in Barker's thinking and, moreover, the stages of appraisal outlined here quickly and farcically escalate so that, clearly, impractical demands are placed on reviewers. Why then detail activities that cannot happen? In response, three points require attention. First, statements to the effect that "all you really need to know is what is the best test to apply in given circumstances" (Barker, 2013, p. 89), statements of the sort widely reproduced in many nursing texts, fail, without explanation, to clarify what is required or involved in meeting this goal. More is rolled into these statements than is commonly realised. Second, through no fault of their own, nurses are ill-equipped to review quantitative studies and 'pushing' what is required in establishing one small facet of warrant exposes this ill-preparedness. Third, if we cannot confidently determine that the best or most appropriate statistical test was used, what sort of review is being conducted? Establishing this thing seems like a minimum requirement. Yet if the steps sketched above are over-elaborate or impractical, how else is this to be done?

Actual calculations and peer review

Regardless of the difficulties encountered above, Barker (ibid.) implicitly acknowledges that we cannot presume researchers always use the best tests. This is why she calls upon reviewers to establish that the best test was picked, and here we agree. However, if it cannot be assumed that the best test 'in theory' is used, why take it for granted that chosen tests are successfully run? As noted, Barker (2013) does not think it "necessary to understand … actual calculations" (p. 89). Yet without this understanding, without being able to work through what occurred, reviewers cannot establish that tests (best or not) are credibly used.

If tests were appropriately run and reported there would be no problem. However, the very opposite can be true (Brown, Kaiser and Allison, 2018). Altman (1994) long ago raised the alarm in regard to medical research (Young, 2007). Yet respected journals continue to publish statistically flawed studies (Cumming, 2014). Mays and Melnyk (2009) suggest that over a third of articles in *Nature* and a quarter of papers in the *British Medical Journal* contain serious statistical errors and/or omissions. Lang (2004) reproduces comments to the effect that half of all biomedical papers contain incorrectly applied statistical methods. Erdmann, De Mast and Warrens (2015) associate methodological with statistical errors. Smaldino and McElreath (2016) highlight the role of misaligned incentives in continuing bad practice. Boutron and Ravaud (2018) discuss the 'spinning' (distortion) of results, and Belluz (2016) claims that "on average – only 3,000 of 50,000 new journal articles published each year are well-designed and relevant enough to inform patient care. That's 6 percent". Moreover, in comments that presumably also apply to nursing, Strasak et al. (2007) state that:

> standards in the use of statistics in medical research are generally low. A growing body of literature points to persistent statistical errors, flaws and deficiencies in most medical journals.
>
> *(Strasak et al., 2007, p. 44)*

These errors include errors of calculation and – to restate – if reviewers do not check actual calculations, they will miss errors and they will accept and possibly act on or utilise results that are incorrect. Reviewers cannot abrogate responsibility. In academic psychology, acknowledgement of this and related problems has and is producing a radical upheaval in the way research is conducted and appraised (Nelson, Simmons and Simonsohn, 2018). Interest in this problem is also apparent in the medical literature (see e.g. Artino et al., 2018; Robinson et al., 2018). However, to date, relatively few nurse methodologists have substantively engaged this subject. Prestigious peer reviewed journals publish unreliable studies (Brembs, 2018), and 'our' journals undoubtedly put out papers containing statistical inaccuracies. Inappropriate tests are therefore used and tests are badly run. When nurse reviewers fail to identify these errors, potentially, patients may be harmed and/or research corrupted. Peer review does not protect or guarantee the warrant of statistically derived findings.

Teamwork – a plan

Returning to the 'tension' in my position referred to earlier, unless reviewers meaningfully understand how findings are concluded then, absent other 'good reason', those findings should not be accepted or acted upon. They remain unwarranted. However, if determining this thing in quantitative research requires that nurses comprehend the statistical tests that were used to formulate findings, then this objective may be beyond the capabilities of many nurses (myself included). Should we then give up reviewing quantitative studies?

This statement and, indeed, arguments presented across the last few pages are deliberately framed in a melodramatic and rigid manner. I take this line because I believe nurses too glibly accept study findings and I want to challenge what I take to be complacency. No doubt my argument is, in places, overly excited. Nonetheless, students and researchers review studies against low epistemic standards, low standards of evaluation correlate with high levels of error acceptance, and care and/or research therefore incorporate and rest on erroneous information. Yet if low standards were to be rejected, we hit the problem of reviewer competence. That is, nurse reviewers are simply not trained to read and understand most of the statistical tests they meet in quantitative studies, these studies cannot then be sensibly appraised, and this reality torpedoes a major element in EBP.

To meet these problems, when reviewing quantitative papers, nurses who lack statistical ability/education might work alongside and with people who do possess these skills. Thus, as in any situation when help is required, 'we' need to cooperate with and seek assistance from others. It may be that these others are not nurses. However, I can think of no reason why they should or must be. Moreover, to force this issue – to ensure the problems outlined here do not pass unnoticed – it might be that journal editors and other key 'gatekeepers' (e.g. research ethics committees, Masters and doctoral supervisors etc.) need to require the higher standards that teamwork is here promoted as enabling. Thus, reviews assessing quantitative reports should not be sanctioned, resourced or accepted for publication or educational accreditation unless reviewers make clear how statistical tests in the papers appraised have been analysed. Further, since this requirement is unlikely to be met by a lone nurse reviewer (or even a small team when that team lacks statistician input) cross- or interdisciplinary working would be necessitated in most and possibly every instance.

Further, in education, the idea that students can and should be able to assess quantitative studies in a meaningful way only makes sense if students are facilitated to engage (at an appropriate level) with the statistical tests reports employ. However, it is likely that most nursing students do not, at present, gain a grounding in statistics commensurate with the requirements made of them and we should therefore ask – what might be done?

Additional to the recommendations made above, first, if it is indeed the case that nurses need to be able to critique quantitative studies in anything other than a trifling manner (and this premise cannot necessarily be assumed), minimally acceptable levels of statistical ability/ competence need to be agreed (my presumption here is that, despite the existence of regulatory and policy guidance, detailed standards on this subject do not exist). Thus, depending on the level at which students and researchers are operating, they and their educators need to know precisely what is expected of them. In my view minimal standards should mandate that reviewers engage with 'actual calculations'. However, as noted, others think differently and this topic requires further extended debate. Second, time and other resources must be allocated to this presently underappreciated and under resourced aspect or element of nurse education. This is problematic. Prioritisation is a (small 'p') political act. When an activity is prioritised, normally, something else is cut or reduced. Thus, if teaching/contact hours are given to statistics, unless the curriculum has spare capacity – which is unlikely – another activity must go or be 'trimmed'. Third, even if agreement was possible on what should be taught, and even if time/resources were available for this endeavour (two very big ifs), given a paucity of statistically literate nurse educators, who should deliver teaching remains open. In some instances, it might be possible for nursing schools and departments, if they cannot access expertise in-house, to recruit or bring in statistical capability from other schools/departments within their institutions and this, to my mind, has the advantage of once more facilitating cross- and interdisciplinary working. Thus, fourth, sourcing non-nursing expertise could enable or play a part in establishing new norms and expectations around review practice. That is, working alongside and with statisticians might be promoted as 'the way' to proceed vis-à-vis quantitative research review. This, I propose, would be a good. Science "is a communal enterprise" (Green, 2018), and peer review is recognised as an effective means of supporting aspects of the review process (Spry and Mierzwinski-Urban, 2018). Yet, reviews are often undertaken by isolated individuals, and ongoing and iterative discussion about methods and outcomes does not always take place. To some degree, teamwork cuts through – potentially – the 'tension' in my position between the need to understand, and difficulty around comprehension. This last proposal will not, however, appeal to nurses who want to bolster and maintain disciplinary boundaries.

Big data and statistical analysis – complication unbound

The problems that nurse reviewers face are further challenged by, among other things, interrelated innovations in quantitative meta-analysis (Liberati et al., 2009), complexity science (Mitchell et al., 2016; Sethi, 2018), evidence mapping (Althuis and Weed, 2013), machine learning (Athey and Imbens, 2015), deep learning (Hughes, 2019), and advanced versions of the hierarchy of evidence – for example, the 5S and now 6S pyramid which moves 'upwards' from studies (primarily experimental randomised controlled trials), to synopses, synthesis, synopses of syntheses, summaries and, finally, systems (Santangelo et al., 2015; Alper and Haynes, 2016; Murad et al., 2016; McMaster University, 2019). These data rich forms of evidence aggregation and presentation can overwhelm the ability of even expert reviewers to meaningfully grasp how conclusions are drawn, and although these techniques and processes are subject to criticism (see e.g. Ioannidis, 2016), nonetheless, huge and disruptive changes in the scale and scope of quantitative data capture and assessment are underway.

The phrase 'big data' has been used to describe this phenomenon, and while the term crudely points towards an array of evolving and converging technologies, computerised processes and organising activities (Lee, 2017), a common thread connecting those involved is the sourcing and interpretation of what, by recent historic standards, are colossal and rapidly expanding amounts of information (Andrew-Perez, et al., 2015; Jain, 2016; Mieronkoski et al., 2017). Commentators such as Few (2018) warn that big data is a fashionable pretender or misnomer insofar as the changes it identifies are incremental and disjointed rather than coherent and revolutionary. Nevertheless, Finlay's (2014) text on predictive analysis, and Witten et al. (2017) on algorithmic data mining, and predictive and descriptive analytics might stand as representative works for the sort of developments being alluded to. That is, they characterise or stand for advances in 'high level' statistical data capture and manipulation and, significantly, these texts address business and commercial audiences. Indeed, big data specialists (for want of a better expression) often operate in spaces outside the academy.

> Increasingly, economic activity turns on collecting and mobilizing information about people. Industries built for this purpose now dwarf the traditional academic departments and think-tanks that once dominated the social sciences. Google … has over 35,000 employees, more than twice the 13,000 academic economists in the United States. And the marketing department of Procter and Gamble is larger than the sociology departments of all US universities combined.
>
> *(Epstein, 2015, p. 2)*

Commercial and state actors have the incentive and resources necessary to invest in and progress forms of data capture and analysis that dwarf or outstrip the capabilities of all but top tier universities or, more accurately, university collaborations. However, as Epstein (2015) notes, the implications of this have yet to be fully realised.

Many of the world's most dynamic enterprises identify data analytics as a core activity, and university teaching and research now often lags behind rather than leads innovation in this field. Thus, across the social sciences, it can no longer be assumed that a university education equips students or researchers to engage at the highest levels with the most advanced methodologies and methods – and universities must, in many instances, learn from rather than educate outsiders. Notably, big data analysts' evidence advanced programming and statistical skills. Collaborative working across professional boundaries is the norm, and modern and costly technical resources are frequently employed. These requirements cut away at the ability of students and researchers operating in segmented, underfunded, and isolated university departments to keep abreast of developments. They pose particular difficulties for nurses.

Gloom aside, Guttmann et al.'s (2011) work positively illustrates what can be achieved when big data is applied to healthcare. This study involved the analysis of 22 million records of patient visits to Ontario (Canada) emergency departments (A&E) over a five-year period. From this data set information on 14 million discharged patients was extracted, and outcome measures for these patients were correlated against average waiting times for attending patients (waiting times here stand as assumed proxies for 'franticness'). Results revealed that:

> as you might fear. For patients sent home who attended an A&E department when the average wait there was more than six hours, the odds of death were almost twice those of patients sent home when the wait was less than one hour. This odds ratio was similar for patients measured as high and low urgency at triage, so it's true for patients with both serious and less serious presentations.
>
> *(Goldacre, 2014b [2011], p. 74)*

Goldacre (2014b [2011]) goes on to note that "even more starkly" (p. 74), analysis indicated that data patterns became "statistically significant when average waits reach just three hours" (p. 74) and, moreover, trends could be seen within as well as between hospitals "so it wasn't just the crap hospitals" (p. 75) that evidenced this relationship.

Interesting as these results are for patients, and one might add, healthcare workers wanting to press for additional resources (though the authors of the report are careful to stress that findings may not be generalisable), their full significance runs beyond any particular case. The example illustrates how the discovery of important but rare events involves locating and analysing vast numbers (millions) of data points. This information can be scattered across multiple platforms. The skills necessary to complete this task are demanding. Extensive teamwork is required and, regrettably, while expertise within the profession is identifiable (see e.g. Murphy, Goossen and Weber, 2017), it is unclear – to put it politely – that many nurses are presently able to participate as equals in this sort of activity (Topaz and Pruinelli, 2017).

On the other hand, is the type of activity described here simply research, or might it be a form of review? I am minded to think that in some instances big data analysis can be classed as a review or, at least, a hybrid review. Guttmann et al.'s (2011) study self-identifies as research (it is a population based retrospective cohort study). Yet it could be argued that the methods used (analysing the contents of computerised health administrative databases) simply expand the definition of literature to include raw data. This statement might seem wrongheaded since, among other criticisms that could be made, the proposed expansion collapses the distinction between primary and secondary source material. However, a great deal of raw data is published or accessible online, it is already the case (previously discussed) that nursing texts on literature searches and reviews treat location and appraisal processes in ways analogous to research and, more significantly, in many respects big data analytics merely reformulate and update techniques currently employed in healthcare meta-analyses and 6S work. That is, forms of quantitative review which already blur the line between research (which creates new data/information) and location-appraisal processes that represent and order (give form to) existing data/information. Thus, while big data exists in diverse forms, it was generated to serve multiple purposes (or none), and it is lodged at manifold locations – meta-analysis, 6S system construction, and big data location-appraisal processes differ in complexity, scale and ambition rather than anything more fundamental. Further, the role and importance of subjective judgement, and the place of the analyst within the interpretation of big data is signalled in, for example, Lowenthal's (2019) work on policy development within the intelligence services and, once more, this configures big data analytics in ways that look a lot like forms of review.

Alternatively, even if we abandon the notion that big data analysis is a type of review, nurses wishing to include the findings of big data research in reviews confront considerable problems. Specifically, for the results of a study to be included in a review, the person or team conducting that review needs to identify and understand the results. Putting to one side problems of identification (health related big data studies may be published in journals not listed in CINAHL), what does understanding involve in this instance?

Reviewers may be aware that big data studies have been concluded on a topic they are investigating. However, if those studies evidence levels of statistical and method complexity that exceed the ability of reviewers to establish warrant (validity, reliability, trustworthiness) – perhaps because the form of computational analysis required involves skills and resources that are untaught and unavailable – those studies can be ignored or, alternatively, abandoning any pretence at critical appraisal, findings may simply be accepted as given. Neither option is appealing. Yet, while problems associated with nurse statistical competence have already been broached, it is important to recognise that the difficulties encountered in reviewing 'a' quantitative study exponentially explode when big data research is considered.

Heavey (2015) suggests that most "nursing students experience a mild sense of panic when they discover they have to take statistics – or any other kind of math for that matter" (p. 2). These comments, which appear towards the beginning of the book *Statistics for Nursing*, pleasingly suggest some nurses are expected to take statistical instruction. Education of this sort is not, however, universally provided, or seen as necessary, and when provided it is unlikely to equip nurses to meet the demands of big data. Indeed, Heavey (2015), who writes for nurses, excuses undergraduate students from the section of her book dealing with regression because this "is a complicated statistical technique" (p. ix). However, the mathematical, statistical and computational ability required to unpick big data and other complex studies dwarfs that required by the types of review more usually undertaken. And while I have argued that nurses should have insight into how findings are derived before they accept and potentially utilise those findings (and I stand by that claim), faced with complex big data work, reviewers who do not work with skilled others may have no option but to accept report findings 'unquestioned'.

Colleagues with whom I work repeatedly state that it is unreasonable and unrealistic to expect that under- and indeed postgraduate students will or should understand the statistical tests that appear in the papers they appraise. My colleagues would 'like' students to comment in written work on the appropriateness of tests used. For example, they would 'like' students to say something along the lines of 'the chi-square (X^2) test is appropriately used in this instance because etc.'. However, even basic statements of this sort are not unanimously seen as obligatory or essential and under- and postgraduate students successfully complete work that, in the review section, contain the briefest of statistical references.

> The purpose of appraising a research study is to identify the strengths and limitations that exist within that work. It is wrong to assume that because something appears in print, or because an author appears well qualified, that the findings will be accurate or that the study was undertaken in a robust manner … [it is] important when reading research to do so with a critical eye and never take what is written at face value.
>
> *(Coughlan and Cronin, 2017, p. 81)*

Methodological texts also, to repeat, vary in how they approach these issues. Coughlan and Cronin's comments are typical of the type of statement made. I read this as implying that, simply put, reviewers are required to reach a judgement about the robustness of whatever study they are reading and, on this basis, they decide whether results are likely to be warranted. The implicit assumption built into this sort of reasoning is that reviewers ought to establish whether results are trustworthy before they consider accepting and 'using' findings, and to this end they need to determine whether studies are appropriately conducted. I have already outlined what this means for me – and Guyatt (1991), who first deployed the phrase evidence-based medicine, rooted the concept in the clinician's ability to critically review and synthesise research findings. This process, in line with my view, places critical review before synthesis. Yet, faced with big data studies, while Djulbegovic and Guyatt (2017) recognise this research offers evidence-based medicine exciting opportunities, and healthcare reviews need to address this thing, establishing research 'robustness' in these instances clearly places Sisyphean burdens on reviewers.

That said, Chapter 5 rejected the idea that excuse is acceptable, and this tough line is maintained here. Excuse is offensive for several reasons. However, most pressingly, as Goh (2017) notes, an "insufficient understanding of statistics means that research studies are vulnerable to statistical manipulation, whether unintentional or otherwise", and, picking up on themes introduced earlier, between "80% and 90% of journal articles have serious flaws in their usage of statistics". These flaws occur in high and low-quality journals, and with the advent and expansion of predatory publishing, the percentage of misleading work is likely to rise rather than fall (Nolfi, Lockhart and Myers, 2015; Oermann et al., 2016; Shamseer et al., 2017).[4] Nurse reviewers must then engage with the robustness of quantitative study designs and/or statistical usage. Too many published studies contain inaccurate findings, complex studies – including big data studies – may include more rather than fewer inaccuracies, and flawed and unwarranted findings should not be allowed to influence practice/research. Nurses therefore confront a choice. Either they abandon attempts to appraise big data quantitative studies (where appraisal cannot escape statistical analysis), or they evaluate studies properly. Here, 'properly' means that sufficient understanding is gained. And while the meaning of sufficient is, of course, open to dispute, it certainly implies something substantive rather than frivolous.

When reviewing quantitative studies, merely determining that the right test was used is not enough. Reviewers also need to establish that it was correctly used. That is, because so many published papers include statistical and computational errors (Choi and Cheung, 2016; Stark and Saltelli, 2018), reviewers ought, in appraisal, to check that findings are correct. Or, alternatively, they need to explain why this was not done/is not required.

This claim is not universally accepted. However, the point here, if these checks are difficult in normal circumstances, they are much more difficult when faced with big data. Attempts to check or appraise these studies require that expert nurse statisticians further 'upskill' and, almost always, teams rather than individuals will be required to tackle this sort of research. Positively, we know patients can benefit from the new informatics (see e.g. Keenan, 2014; Glenn, 2016; Risling, 2017), and some nurses show interest in the subject (Bickford, 2017; O'Conner, 2018). However, concerns are expressed regards big data in nursing (Milton, 2017); and nurse educators, myself included, are woefully underprepared to grapple with the issues involved. We introduce review appraisal skills to students *as if* this activity could and should be performed by individuals rather than collaborative cross- and inter-disciplinary teams. And heedless of external developments, nursing departments continue to train quantitative researchers – including Masters and doctoral candidates – in methods that are positively antediluvian when compared alongside those outlined by, for example, Finlay (2014) and Witten et al. (2017).

Why this problem?

Backwardness in part references what Glaister (2007) terms computer anxiety among nursing students and, we might suppose, nurses more generally. It also, to repeat, reflects the poor mathematical and statistical ability of many nurses (Harvey et al., 2010; Eastwood et al., 2011). Thus, despite acknowledged importance (Sandwell and Carson, 2005; Hayat et al., 2013), substantive mathematical and/or statistical education is rarely offered in undergraduate programmes and, for example, instruction may fail to progress beyond the simplest discussion of easily misused-misinterpreted P values (Nuzzo, 2014; Briggs, 2017; Spurlock, 2017; Ziliak, 2017). It is hardly surprising then that nurses find it difficult to utilise statistics in academic and/or clinical practice (Gaudet, 2014; MyoungJin and Hayat, 2015). This much is known. However, further, it may be that the lack of mathematical and statistical acumen among nurses is aggravated – it might not be helped – by recruitment strategies which prioritise expressed values over academic ability (see e.g. Miller, 2015; Newton et al., 2015; Kirman, 2016; Patterson et al., 2016; Scammell, 2016; Tetley et al., 2016).

Values based recruitment has been mandated in the UK since 2015 (Mazhindu et al., 2016), and while putative students are encouraged to prepare themselves for interview so that they evince appropriate other regarding attitudes (see e.g. Day-Calder, 2017), the need to display critical thinking, intellectual and/or significant mathematical-statistical ability at interview is not similarly accented.[5] Sharon and Grinberg (2018) suggest that high levels of emotional intelligence are associated with degree success, and they propose that emotional intelligence ought to be assessed upon admission. However, this form of intelligence (if that is the right word) need not correlate with or represent the type of ability that, I suggest, is underplayed in recruitment and, arguably, this entrenches the idea that nurses should be 'nice' rather than 'clever'. Indeed, in downplaying intellectual achievement, fresh credence is perhaps given to the notion that nurses educated to degree level lack compassion and/or are 'too posh to wash' (Rolfe, 2015; Aubeeluck, Stacey and Stupple, 2016).

The 'nice vs. clever' dichotomy takes many forms and, for example, while Henderson and Jones (2017) rightly emphasise the importance of compassion in care, overemphasising values might displace or deprioritise the role of intelligence in nursing. There is, it must be stressed, nothing intrinsically oppositional between niceness and cleverness. Nonetheless, it is noticeable that while, for example, O'Grady et al. (2017) quite reasonably state that "People expect to receive nursing care from compassionate, caring and committed professionals" (p. 47) – 'people' do not apparently automatically expect to receive care from knowledgeable or skilled (let alone mathematically or statistically competent) nurses. Indeed, in recruitment and also in nursing's literature, being well intentioned and kind seem, sometimes, to take precedence over proficiency and expertise.

It may be that I here misrepresent authors who, for perfectly good reasons, underscore the importance of compassion. Nonetheless, highlighting values without simultaneously promoting intelligence suggests intelligence is less valued. This gives the impression that either intelligent people are not compassionate, or compassion does not require or involve intelligently grounded action (i.e. it is enough to emote). This is odd. Research suggests that the quality of care is – unsurprisingly – associated with the intelligence/education of caregivers (Kutney-Lee, Sloane and Aiken, 2013; Aiken et al., 2014; Rafferty, 2018; see also Chapter 1). Yet this association is rarely articulated in compassion dialogues. And, while the significance of competence is recognised, and competence can substitute for skill (Baillie, 2017), the requirement that nurses display an aptitude for technical or intellectual capability (or indeed critical thinking/creativity, Dyson, 2018) receives comparatively little attention in values-based recruitment strategies. Further, within the methodological literature, the idea that reviews (supposedly an essential or core nursing skill – Lipp and Fothergill, 2015; Moule, 2018) might require significant intellectual ability from reviewers is similarly (and strangely) downplayed. Reticence regards what is involved is difficult to fathom. However, if an 'essential' skill (i.e. one all should possess) places demands on practitioners that not all practitioners can realistically or substantively meet, awkward questions concerning the suitability of candidates and/or practitioners are generated.

Exceptionalism, defensiveness, irrationalism

Cohn, Jia and Larson (2009) argue that interdisciplinary authorship and a statistician co-author were predictive of high-quality quantitative studies in nursing journals and, one might add, teamwork of this sort is intuitively beneficial in reviews. Thus, Rojas et al.'s (2016) paper on data process mining in healthcare notably involved contributors from computer science, engineering, and medicine. Big data and data science is, as noted, inherently cross- and inter-disciplinary in scope. Big data, for example, complements advances in behavioural psychology, and a great deal of new thinking in psychology popularised by, amongst others, Thaler and Sunstein (2009), Sutherland (2013), Sunstein (2015) and Tetlock and Gardner (2016), derives its power and influence from the creation and exploitation of large data sets by interdisciplinary teams. I do not know how people active in these fields would react to Aveyard, Payne and Preston's (2016, p. 52) assertion that a discipline should only engage with theories "relevant to your academic discipline" (see Chapter 1). However, since many of the theories (models, concepts, ideas) driving big data work defy disciplinary categorisation, I suspect responses would include astonishment and derision.[6]

This matters. If cross-disciplinary activity and the boundary fluidity this encourages is perceived as threatening, nurses may be reluctant to work with and learn from non-nurses. In the Preface, defensiveness was linked with the idea of professional exceptionalism. Thus, if nurses believe they possess a unique and ethically privileged position or vantage within healthcare, when it is thought that 'we' care in special (holistic) ways that are unavailable to others, and if it is assumed that the nursing profession needs to be bolstered and protected (see e.g. Hanucharurnkul and Turale, 2017; Parse, 2017), exceptionalism acts to block cross- and inter-disciplinary working. After all, how can 'we' function as equals alongside others in using big data methodologies and methods when 'they' lack crucial insights only 'we' possess?

> As we move the profession forward with advanced degrees and different skill sets, it is extremely important that we project a positive image. That image is seen by others, not only in our appearance and attitudes, but in the way we communicate. Each individual nurse practitioner is a representative of the profession. An individual cannot separate 'self' from the profession or the organization to which they belong.
>
> *(Watkins, 2015, p. 1)*

Watkins' (2015) proclamation in the Mississippi Nurses Association 'Report from Council on Advanced Practice' is not about big data. However, it evidences the defensiveness that is intrinsic to exceptionalist conceptions of nursing. Here, despite mention of advanced degrees (i.e. progress in nursing's professional project), it is important (why?) that nurses project a positive image to 'others' (who? of what?). Moreover, in this projection, nurses are not individuals. Rather, they are members of a collective exhibiting group identity. This, we are gnomically told, "is the secret knowledge that demonstrates the continuation of a profession" (p. 1). Further, while this (circa 2015) "is an exciting time" it is also "a very concerning time" and "We must be mindful" not to "jeopardize our progress. We are under the microscope, our every action will be examined. We must be careful in the words we write that are viewed by others" (p. 1).

Watkins' vision of nursing is distrustful. She fears 'others' who wish to do nursing down, and she worries about nurses least they betray whatever it is that needs protecting. It might be objected that I here unfairly pick on a short opinion piece. However, the example was chosen because of its essential blandness. Watkins presents us with a mild illustration of exceptionalism-defensiveness. Large numbers of similar and more extreme commentaries populate 'our' literature, and defensiveness grounded in exceptionalism is a widespread phenomenon.

Exceptionalism also lends itself to irrationalism and mystical occultism (Watkins' 'secret knowledge'). After all, since only 'we' care in 'our' special nursing (holistic) way, and since anyone can be trained to perform technical tasks, it cannot be the technical or reductive which marks out nursing. Arguably, the profession's apparent willingness to sanction discussion of homeopathy (Schulenburg, 2015; Hamilton, 2016) and/or therapeutic touch "defined as an intervention derived from the laying on of hands. The hands help to transfer energy from a person serving as a healer to another person" (Coakley, Barron and Annese, 2016), signal these influences. And while Glazer (2001) demolishes energies nonsense, and the European Academies Science Advisory Council (EASAC, 2017) refute homeopathy, these and other scatty ways of envisioning care continue to find a place in the nursing literature.

Exceptionalist pretensions and a warped understanding of holism lie behind, in my view, commentaries on, for example, prayer (see e.g. Ameling, 2000; Holt-Ashley, 2000; Perry, 2005; Narayanasamy and Narayanasamy, 2008), and pliable interpretations of spirituality sanction discussion of naturopathy, craniosacral therapy, energy realignment, and much more wackiness besides. For those who are interested, *Visions* the journal of Rogerian Nursing

Science is worth consulting here (www.societyofrogerianscholars.org/index.html). And Phillips (2017) "theory of pandimensional awareness-integral presence … [where] The relation of wellbecoming and integral presence contributes to the theory, as well as discussion of human field image and human field hugs" (p. 223), is suggestive of what can be sourced.

Summation

Quantitative investigation generates knowledge that productively informs patient care and further research. However, some and possibly most nurse reviewers find it difficult to substantively interpret the tests used in generating results. Problems can be overblown. A great many successful reviews are completed. Nonetheless, when reviewers cannot establish how conclusions are derived, when they do not meaningfully comprehend the tests employed in producing results, since 'warrant' remains indeterminate, those findings ought not to be accepted or acted on. Others will disagree. However, those who demur should perhaps state their reasons and this, I suggest, may prove difficult to do.

Under- and postgraduate nursing students, educators and early career researchers are often ill prepared (they are not educated) to engage in or with serious mathematical modelling and statistical analysis. Where lack of preparation hampers the review of 'normal' quantitative studies, it is highly likely that developing forms of complex statistical research (here defined as 'big data') remain beyond comprehension.

Cross and inter-disciplinary teamwork is suggested as one means by which the sorts of problem identified here (including 'tensions' in my position) might be met. However, a profession which valorises values above intelligence, a profession that is distrustful and defensive in its interactions with others, a profession in which anagonical, mystical and irrationalist thinking finds leg room, is unlikely to seek common ground or purpose with disciplines engaged in sophisticated data analytics. Getting to grips with statistics is not then simply an educational or technical issue. Rather, thinking about why nurses and nursing have difficulty with these issues highlight aspects of professionalism (and the critique of professionalism) that reviewers ought possibly to consider.

Notes

1 It is thus assumed that only warranted research results should inform practice and/or review conclusions (research). However, not only can this position be disputed (see e.g. Pawson, 2006) but what counts as 'warrant' requires, possibly, greater elaboration. Placing the explanation offered in this chapter alongside Price's (1967) work on knowing and believing suggests, for example, that warrant is a more nuanced concept than is here allowed. Further, as reference to Clifford (2018 [1877] – see Chapter 2) suggests, beliefs that are influenced even triflingly (perhaps in response to reading a partially understood research paper) are likely to have or evince consequences.

2 Not every quantitative study aims at producing generalisable findings. Nonetheless, generalisability is a key facet or claimed benefit of randomised control trial findings. When performed successfully, it is generally supposed that experimental studies provide generalisable knowledge (Bench, Day and Metcalfe, 2013; Ingham-Broomfield, 2016). And while EBP rests on more than quantitative research (Rycroft-Malone et al., 2004; Greenhalgh, 2018), the existence of generalisable findings grounded on inductive and deductive statistical models contributes to the idea that at least some nursing actions have a solid or defendable evidence base (Flemming, 2007b). Generalisability is a property or outcome of certain forms of (causal) statistical inference (Bareinboim, 2014), and quantification, generalisability and statistics are closely conjoined. That said, statistical generalisation is a sprawling and

complex concept – and key elements of the construct remain disputed (Lee and Baskerville, 2003; Fendler, 2006; Lee and Baskerville, 2012; Tsang and Williams, 2012; Hohmann et al., 2018).

3 National Institute for Health and Care Excellence – www.nice.org.uk/

4 Predatory or exploitative 'for-profit' journals raise a host of tricky issues for reviewers. Since robust peer-review processes have not been followed it might, for example, be assumed that material in these journals should be ignored. However, just as nonsense is published in reputable journals, so informative and useful papers may appear in otherwise worthless publications and – to state the obvious – if these 'good' papers are identifiable, they might be judged relevant sources.

5 It would be difficult to argue that the maths test which accompanies recruitment is in any sense demanding.

6 Hughes (2019) similarly argues that extensive team and cross-disciplinary coordination between data scientists and healthcare workers is required when complex statistical tests are employed.

7

REVIEWING QUALITATIVE RESEARCH

- Consensus is absent on whether the quality of qualitative research can or even should be assessed.
- If agreement on how the quality of qualitative studies are to be evaluated does not exist, the results of these studies cannot but sit awkwardly within the standard model of reviews.
- The non-generalisability of qualitative research findings remains a problem for reviewers.
- The theoretical underpinnings of qualitative synthesis remain underdeveloped.
- It is suggested that the quality of qualitative synthesis can be poor or indeterminate.
- To meet some of the difficulties encountered in defending (and therefore using) qualitative results, researchers should perhaps be encouraged to implement active citation.

While the evaluation of quantitative research presents difficulties for reviewers, qualitative appraisal is, arguably, even more challenging. A veritable cottage industry exists on and around determining the quality and evidential worth of qualitative studies (see e.g. Flick, 2008; Collingridge and Gantt, 2008; Shenton, 2004; Tracy, 2010; Thorne, 2016a; and Welch and Piekkari, 2017). However, despite this expenditure of effort, commentators continue to disagree on issues as fundamental as whether the quality of qualitative studies can or even should be assessed.

> There is considerable debate around the quality assessment of qualitative research as to whether it can, or indeed should be done. There is little consensus on how quality assessment should be undertaken within qualitative research with over a hundred sets of proposals on quality in qualitative research ... and widely opposing views on the matter. ... There is further contention about how best to approach quality assessment given evidence that it cannot be performed reliably.
>
> *(Booth, Papaioannou and Sutton, 2012, p. 113)*

No consensus

The standard model of review procedure assumes that good rather than bad quality studies will be included in reviews. Common sense also demands that the soundness of studies be assessed since to abandon this possibility rescinds or annuls the very idea of meaningful evaluation. Indeed, if reviewers are unable to reach defendable judgements about the quality of studies and the robustness or worth of findings then, perhaps, all that remains is the uncritical and passive acceptance of whatever researchers say.

That said, while reviewers want to determine the quality of qualitative studies, Booth, Papaioannou and Sutton (2012) problematise this ambition. Specifically, they advance three distinct claims, the importance of which cannot be overemphasised. First, it is asserted that debate as to whether qualitative research can and should be assessed is unresolved and ongoing. Second, they note that little consensus exists regarding how, if it should, evaluation ought to proceed. Third, it is recognised that even when undertaken, appraisal may be unreliable. It is not necessary here to become embroiled in substantiating and/or critiquing these propositions (readers can easily access literature on these subjects, and relevant sources are cited throughout this chapter). Rather, whatever position one adopts vis-à-vis these claims, it is the lack of consensus that matters.

Chapter 6 noted that although statistical tests are tough to interpret, in principle – following education – it is or should be possible to determine that appropriate tests are used and (if sufficient detail is provided) successfully run. That is, widespread if not universal agreement on this subject is feasible. However, when it comes to the assessment of qualitative work, Booth, Papaioannou and Sutton's (2012) comments undermine the idea that consensus is obtainable. Claims to the effect that agreement on the quality of qualitative work cannot be established cut away at the place and role of such studies in practice or research. Yet, as noted, very large numbers of 'guides' exist, so why not pick and utilise one of these?

For argument's sake, let us suppose that at least some of the hundred plus proposals regarding qualitative appraisal permit studies to be differentiated according to quality. This possibility is contestable but, also, plausible. Regrettably allowing that some critiquing tools or frameworks may enable the quality of qualitative studies to be assessed does not release nurse reviewers from their bind since, even if evaluation is viable, without an agreed comparator metric – i.e. absent defendable agreement – how reviewers are to sift this jumble of approaches remains unresolved. We simply do not know how to identify effective tools and frameworks.

Thus, presumably tools and frameworks vary in effectiveness. Some are almost certainly useless. Yet without consensus on what 'good' qualitative research does or looks like, reviewer choices about critiquing guides appear disquietingly arbitrary. That is, you could pick tool or framework 'x' and I might pick 'y', and although we might review the same paper, potentially we could reach different conclusions regards quality ignorant of or indifferent to our respective choices. It hardly matters. There is no way of establishing which review is best/better since we do not know what best means and, further, even where 'an' approach to reviewing is agreed upon (i.e. even when we both adopt method 'x'), because tools/frameworks are interpreted rather than applied, the reliability of reviews derived from 'an' approach cannot be independently verified.

> Review authors engaged in qualitative evidence synthesis may take radical philosophical positions towards quality assessment that sometimes oppose each other … qualitatively oriented review authors would argue that the focus on limiting bias to establish validity

is antithetical to the philosophical foundations of qualitative approaches to inquiry.... The researcher is the instrument through which data are collected and analyzed. Consequently, the data analysis is legitimately influenced by the researchers when they interpret the data.... A second group of qualitative review authors promotes the principle that qualitative research studies should be assessed using the same criteria as used in appraising quantitative research, that is, the quality of original research should first of all be evaluated in terms of their ability to produce valid, reliable, and generalizable research findings.

(Hannes, 2017, p. 136)

Confronting the issue identified by Booth, Papaioannou and Sutton (2012), Hannes (2017) sketches two contrasting styles of qualitative research synthesis and adds "ongoing debates on what constitutes quality in research and which criteria to opt for in the assessment of quantitative and qualitative studies show that quality is a multi-dimensional concept" (p. 138). This may well be true. Quality might be multi-dimensional. Yet this is unlikely to satisfy or meet the needs of nurses seeking clarification on how to appraise qualitative work. This admission merely points the way to hyper complexity and aggravated disagreement.

Synthesis is examined shortly. However, before then, a few more words must be said about the evaluation of individual studies and, thus, while qualitative research assumes a bewildering variety of forms, and homogeneity within this methodology must not be overegged (Creswell, 1998; Freeman, 2006), qualitative research of the sort published in nursing journals frequently references the idea that 'themes emerge from data', and this key concept requires brief attention.

Emergence, rhetoric, and warrant

Although the descriptor is beginning to lose favour, it remains the case that qualitative researchers (in texts accessed by students) frequently assert that themes emerge from and hence exist within data. This claim – this use of the concept 'emergence' – is challenged by, among others, Paley (2017). His proposals refer to particular forms of qualitative research. Nonetheless, this feature of his argument applies widely.

I read Paley as suggesting that qualitative researchers do not mine data to extract themes. That is, researchers are not uncovering or digging out what lays buried, and emergent themes are not hidden nuggets. Rather, researchers are the lens through which interpretations are shaped. And, moreover, the background assumptions and theories that researchers wittingly and unwittingly hold form the suspensory ligaments or extra-ocular muscles that focus the researcher's gaze. This metaphor leads us to see emergence as a reference for informed and imaginative researcher judgement. That is, researchers 'find' meaning in texts only insofar as they creatively identify meaning. A vital concept and literary trope in qualitative work, emergence describes the process through which findings are derived, and sticking with the idea first outlined in Chapter 6 that reviewers need to comprehend and assess how results are derived before those findings can be accepted and used, it can be supposed – to some extent – that emergence plays an analogous role to that served by statistical tests in quantitative work.

In contrast to statistical tests, however, the way in which emergence takes place remains underexplained and, perhaps, it is unexplainable. Labels are attached to the stages of emergence or thinking, and readers are thus told that codes, categories and such like are identified. Yet because the researcher is the interpretive tool (Hannes, 2017), and since we cannot see inside researcher heads, even comprehensive explanations of emergence do not fully capture what is involved. Further, this failure in explanation is inevitable. Many and perhaps most of the thought processes that contribute to meaning attribution may be invisible to or unrealised by those doing the attributing (here researchers),[1] and qualitative findings might, in vital respects, therefore be conceptualised as assertions. That is, regardless of the amount or level of detail provided, researchers ultimately assert that, in their considered opinion, 'this' interpretation is to be preferred. To give order and credibility to interpretation the language of emergence (codes, categories, *etc.*) is used. Nevertheless, while these terms lend qualitative studies an air of objectivity, stripped of jargon, qualitative researchers simply declare that the themes they identify best describe, in their opinion, what others said and/or experienced. However, rather than saying 'on these grounds, this is my interpretation' we are told that 'themes emerged'.

Not, I hasten to add, that there is anything wrong with interpretation or the subjective judgement it incorporates. This is only a problem if we assume qualitative research is an aspect of science, and science is or should be objective and/or value free. Further, looking beyond nursing, while numerous theories of, for example, history and historical writing exist (Gardiner, 1959; Bloch, 1976 [1954]), almost without exception these theories recognise and value subjective judgement in the interpretation of facts-evidence. Historians are not embarrassed by this. They rely on judgement in narrative constructions that are evidence informed but not value free. And the impact of subjective influence is likewise documented in traditional laboratory science (Harré, 2009). Interpretations offered in qualitative studies thus weave empiric data and subjective judgement together. Done well, what is concluded can be inspiring, interesting, and important (see Chapter 2). However, deciding when qualitative studies are 'done well' is, as Booth, Papaioannou and Sutton (2012) ably state, highly problematic, and the language of emergence obfuscates rather than illuminates what happens during interpretation. That is, by describing coding strategies in mechanistic ways that allude to scientific processes rather than informed but creative explanation, reviewers can be misled.

Determining how qualitative results are derived is therefore difficult. Most published reports (at least those in mainstream or 'popular' nursing journals) provide insufficient explanatory detail and, also, because interpretation occurs inside the head of researchers, in almost every instance it is impossible to accurately and robustly describe the logic or chains or reasoning involved in establishing results. Not that this is obvious. Qualitative research reports, like all research reports, aim to persuade. And reviewers are encouraged to think they comprehend what is going on.

Researchers thus work to convince readers (here reviewers) that their interpretations are trustworthy, and a great deal of effort goes into choosing participant quotations and theme headings that convey the right impression (Mitchell and Clark, 2018). There is nothing wrong with this. Rhetoric and rhetorical skill are integral to argument, and stylistic device cannot be removed from communication (written and verbal) without crippling the ability of communication to carry meaning. However, that said, qualitative papers can arouse strong emotional responses in readers, and while such responses may be inevitable or inescapable, affect is evidence only for affect (Hempel, 1945). That is, sentiment and the accuracy (or otherwise) of findings bear no necessary relation. We can be duped into feeling strongly about claims that prove to be palpably untrue (or vacuous), and basing belief solely on psychological rather than logical or empiric grounds is rarely recommended. Put simply, while we might be profoundly 'moved' by what is said, emotive reaction and the correctness of what is proposed are or can be different things (this statement does not contradict arguments presented in Chapter 4). Further, while rhetorical and other persuasive devices are used by researchers (and, to repeat, they run through all communication), a great deal hangs on linguistic performance in qualitative reports. That is, the trustworthiness of qualitative findings is conveyed as much by skilful writing as by data presentation, and this distinguishes qualitative from quantitative research where, ultimately, numbers count. In this qualitative writing evinces strong affinities with humanistic scholarship.

Responding to these statements, social constructionists, constructivists, and others, might object that 'accuracy', 'truth' and 'correctness' are inappropriate terms to use in relation to qualitative interpretative work. After all, 'a' construal of evidence does not exhaust those that might be made, and/or these terms might be thought unfitting when applied to descriptions of subjective experience. However, if qualitative researchers are not prepared to stand by their findings, if findings really are just 'an' interpretation, if researchers grant that other interpretations are or could be equally good (whatever that means), or better (ditto), why should a reviewer read and appraise that work? Other than amusement, what would be the point?

Presuming that qualitative researchers intend to say something substantive about whatever it is they investigated, we are stuck with the problem that interpretative processes (i.e. identifying emergent themes) are 'internal' psychological affairs. Justifications (rationales) will be provided for the interpretation offered, and these can be convincing. However, arguments presented in support of findings (interpretation) can never fully convey the processes involved. Reviewers cannot then determine how findings are derived in a full or comprehensive sense. And if reviewers need to meaningfully understand how findings are concluded before they accept and act on those findings, if this is an element in establishing warrant or trustworthiness (see Chapter 6), then without comprehending derivation, those findings cannot sensibly inform practice or influence or contribute to other research.

This is, I appreciate, a radical position. Nonetheless, if rejected, are we saying reviewers can legitimately accept findings on the basis of the arguments and information contained in qualitative research reports? In the nursing literature it is common for published papers to be capped at 5,000 words or less. Do we honestly think researchers can adequately explain and demonstrate the richness of data, the complexity of what is described, and comprehensively outline the interpretive process involved within such a constricted frame? If not, surely reviewers are being asked to accept asserted conclusions on the authority of researcher say so.[2] Or, alternatively, if it is a mistake to require that reviewers comprehend how findings are derived before those findings are accepted, is it being claimed there is something about overall argument that establishes warrant or trustworthiness? And, if it is persuasiveness that matters, should we treat and evaluate qualitative reports as humanities rather than scientific products?

I do not have answers to these puzzles. However, nurse reviewers face complex conundrums when they attempt to evaluate the quality of qualitative studies, and it is difficult not to suppose that – like other facets of the review process – it is easier to ignore than deal with these problems.

Generalisability and the standard model

Agreement on if and how qualitative studies can be appraised is absent, and the ability of reviewers to understand how findings are derived can be disputed. That said, since qualitative studies focus on questions of value and meaning, it might be argued that they meet the needs or requirements of what, in Chapter 2, I called non-scientific questions. This is correct, but only in part. How then do qualitative studies fit within the standard model?

Positively, qualitative studies are – to repeat – often stimulating and illuminating (Greenhalgh, 2018). They can reframe or reconfigure existing understandings, and they can overturn misconceptions. As Guba and Lincoln (1998) note, qualitative data provide "rich insight into human behaviour" (p. 198). However, because "there is no consensus for assessing any piece of qualitative research work" (Leung, 2015, p. 325), the task of excluding poor quality qualitative studies from reviews is complicated. Moreover, even if good quality qualitative studies are identified (and I remain baffled by what 'good' means methodologically in this context), widespread agreement exists to the effect that this form of study does not produce generalisable results (see e.g. Miers, 2000; Freshwater, 2004; Parahoo, 2006; Polit and Beck, 2010; Setia, 2017). The term is attached to qualitative work (see e.g. Miles and Huberman, 1994; Thomas, 2011), and generalising claims are made on the basis of qualitative studies when, for example, recommendations for practice are derived from qualitative findings (Newell and Burnard, 2006), or the meaning of generalisation is reconfigured (Brett, 2018). However, the relevance or use value of qualitative findings in clinical contexts remains indeterminate (Tracy, 2010; Lipscomb, 2012a; 2012b), and when combined in reviews, it is not at all clear what is going on.

Thus, despite arguments favouring expanding the meaning of generalisation and/or launching other claims regards the transferability (rather than generalisability) of qualitative findings (see e.g. Horsburgh, 2003; Eisenhart, 2009; Morse, 2015; van Wijngaarden, Meide and Dahlberg, 2017), these studies do not meet natural science criteria for external validity (Seale, 1999), and they do "not offer evidence of effectiveness in the way that quantitative research does" (Broom, Mahoney and Sellman, 2017, p. 215). Further, since qualitative findings are non-generalisable against statistical or 'Windelbandian' (Lamiell, 1998) nomothetic criteria, anyone attempting to include qualitative studies within a review aligned to the standard model confronts a difficulty. Specifically, reviews are conducted to 'answer' questions, and unless reviewers stipulate that they are interested in, for example, questions related to the perceptions (thoughts, feelings, experiences) of tiny numbers of purposefully chosen and unrepresentative (unique) participants, it is not clear how or in what manner this objective (answering a question) is met by qualitative study findings. Phrasing the problem in this way is intentionally confrontational. Obviously, qualitative reports can, to repeat, be immensely stirring, we can take a lot from them. However, what they tell us, and the epistemological status of that knowledge, sits uneasily within standard model review protocols that seek to guide action by, to repeat, answering questions.

Synthesis, generalisability, and sophistication

The standard model of reviews requires that reviewers set an answerable question. Relevant evidence (usually research papers) are then located, appraised, and 'findings' are thereafter synthesised in order that, hopefully, the initiating question is resolved. Perhaps then the difficulties described above are resolved by or through synthesis?

Qualitative research is noticeably absent from widely used hierarchies of evidence (see e.g. SIGN, 2014), and qualitative studies are infrequently combined in high status reviews (the first synthesis of qualitative evidence was not published by *The Cochrane Database of Systematic Reviews* until 2013). Nonetheless, positively, synthesis would – if it creates or allows for generalisation – provide qualitative research with a place on the upper rungs of the hierarchy of evidence (Flemming, 2007a). Techniques for combining qualitative research are advanced by many scholars (see e.g. Greenhalgh, 2004; Lockwood, 2015; Mohammed, Moles and Chen, 2016) and one or more of these techniques may prove successful. That is, if we ignore worries articulated by Booth, Papaioannou and Sutton (2012) concerning the determination of quality, as well as anxieties around the ability of reviewers to comprehend finding derivation, and the epistemic status of qualitative claims, it might be possible to productively blend the findings of individual qualitative reports together.

> Single qualitative investigations are not intended to produce findings that are directly applicable to clinical practice.
>
> *(Finfgeld-Connett, 2010, p. 246)*

However, if discrete study findings are not 'applicable' in practice, and if qualitative results are non-generalisable, what is changed by aggregation (synthesis)? What occurs during the assessment and combination of non-generalisable qualitative results that transmutes those results into something generalisable? If such alchemy occurs, I have yet to see this convincingly argued. Or, perhaps, qualitative synthesis does not produce generalising claims – except it always does. What other purpose does synthesis have?

Nonetheless, putting these concerns to one side, reviewers choosing to amalgamate qualitative findings must deploy considerable sophistication, and if published studies are a guide to go by, successful combination is not always achieved (Thorne et al., 2004). Indeed, in an indictment of the ability of nurses to combine the findings of qualitative studies in review syntheses, it is alleged that there has been an increase in submissions for publication of perfunctory:

> "quick and dirty" technical reports that position themselves as products of "qualitative metasynthesis." In keeping with the more typical convention that has become popular in evidence synthesis reporting, they focus considerable effort on search, retrieval, and selection decisions, including the deployment of rather arbitrary "quality checklists," such that the majority of available qualitative publications are generally excluded from their final data set. From there, they tend to report superficial findings comprised of thematic similarities, rarely tapping into anything of interest relative to methodological, theoretical, or contextual variance within the selected set of studies. Although they often cite classic qualitative metasynthesis methods references as their analytic resource, the final products of these exercises reflect very little by way of inductive analysis or interpretive examination.
>
> *(Thorne, 2017, p. 3)*

Sally Thorne is editor-in-chief of the journal *Nursing Inquiry*, and this gives weight to her comments regards publishing trends. Many factors contribute to the problems identified in the preceding quotation. However, from the range of issues in play, theoretic complexity and the positioning of syntheses within frameworks that prioritise action over contemplation require special attention.

As noted, the standard model directs reviewers to produce "recommendations for practice" (Aveyard, 2018, p. 4) and to this end, introductory and advanced methodological texts require that defined, precise, and bounded questions – in essence, answerable questions – be framed. This can make sense. Researchers want to efficiently locate the papers that best situate and inform their work, and it is quite reasonable to anticipate that clinicians need to find research reports and other documents that, post-review, identify evidence capable of underpinning action in the world. For reviewers, any lack of clarity in defining the goal of a search may lead to or encourage the use of incoherent and disparately muddled search terms which, unavoidably, cannot but generate randomly meaningless hits (garbage in, garbage out).

Further, EBP's exponents assert that some forms of research finding (e.g. randomised controlled trial data) can directly support clinical behaviour. That is, it is assumed that professionals go to the literature primarily seeking warranted guidance and it is on this basis, on the promise that research findings can influence practice, that EBP is sold to nurses. Thus, while the complex set of concepts and practices that constitute EBP can be articulated and interpreted in various ways, EBP is frequently positioned as a means of informing decision making. From this standpoint EBP is a tool that connects objective research results with clinical questions (through the prism of expressed patient wants/needs and professional insight) in order that those questions can be answered and, hence, defensible action taken. Posing answerable questions and seeking out particular forms of research is seen as crucial in enabling this.

On occasion – and more often than might be supposed – this ideal is realised. EBP works (Green et al., 2014; Brown, 2015). Yet searches and reviews regularly reveal that more or better findings are needed before robust and secure answers can be formulated. This commonly encountered problem frustrates researchers keen to explore and test their own ideas, as well as clinicians anxious to discover the 'correct' way to proceed. Recognising gaps in knowledge undercuts confidence, and though it may be an awkward truth, acknowledging that nurses sometimes act in the absence of evidence (i.e. a firm rationale) destabilises claims to professional expertise. Nevertheless, regardless of whether valid and reliable research findings exist or not, investigating what might be termed answerable questions relies on literature which, conceptual opacity notwithstanding, is scientific, empiric and – generally – quantitative in character.

This claim, first introduced in Chapter 1, problematises the place of qualitative work in reviews. Thorne's (2017) comments (above) suggest nursing meta-syntheses are not always done well, and part of the reason for this involves the use of checklists that, I suggest, ape quantitative practices and 'logics'. Qualitative reports can encourage and inspire fresh thinking. However, this contemplative dimension or potential rubs uneasily against the more action orientated latency of quantitative results. That is, arguably, while qualitative findings facilitate introspection and thought, quantitative generalisation informs concrete action. Where then do qualitative studies fit within the scientific and non-scientific question dichotomy outlined previously?

Science and synthesis

The standard model relies on a restricted and restricting notion of empiric research. However, nailing down what science and scientific methods include and exclude is no simple task, and explanations moving beyond banalities might talk to and juxtapose constructionism, deconstructionism, idealism, interpretivism, naturalism, positivism, post-positivism, realism *etcetera* (this list is easily extendable).

Given this marketplace of ideas, it is perhaps unsurprising that incendiary quarrels around the placing and policing of science's frontiers endure and continue to flare up (Hitchcock, 2004; Achinstein, 2010; Salmon, 2013 [1992]; Chomsky, 2014; Risjord, 2014; Garrett, 2018). In healthcare, these quarrels assume a variety of guises and, for example, while the precise nature, basis, and use value of evidence is, regardless of form, contentious (Rolfe et al., 2008; Greenhalgh and Russel, 2009 – see also Achinstein, 2001), with regard to EBP and nursing, the credentials and epistemic worth of certain types of phenomenological study remain something of a hot potato (Barkway, 2001; McNamara, 2005; Petrovskaya, 2014; Paley, 2017). Moreover, it is suggested that, more generally, qualitative findings cannot be "meaningfully construed as *evidence*" (Thorne, 2016b, p. 157 – italicisation in original), and while this comment is strongly phrased (perhaps too strongly), Paley (2016), who is prepared to grant the title of evidence to qualitative work, nonetheless persuasively argues that the "claim that qualitative research evidence should be placed on an equal footing with experimental and statistical evidence is … quite without warrant" (p. 146).

Like Paley (2016), I think qualitative findings can be evidence. However, as discussed, acknowledged difficulties in assessing the quality of qualitative work and the non-generalisable nature of findings present reviewers with obvious and well-rehearsed puzzles (Dixon-Woods et al., 2004; Hammersley, 2007; Leung, 2015). Moreover, despite claims that "all types of literature" (Aveyard, 2014, p. 67), including qualitative studies, can be included in reviews, the means by which this might be achieved remain contested. Part of the difficulty here is that:

> qualitative research is complex to combine in a review as there are different philosophical underpinnings to the different qualitative methods used and there is the risk of loss of context if these approaches are combined.
>
> *(Aveyard, Payne and Preston, 2016, p. 22)*

Quantitative research can also rest on contrasting philosophic perspectives, and combining findings from these studies raises its own set of questions. Yet, having noted this underpinning problem in regard to qualitative synthesis, Aveyard, Payne and Preston (2016) do not develop it.

The loss of context that occurs when qualitative findings are compared and combined outside the unique situations in which those findings are generated is undeniably important. Context in qualitative study is integral to the derivation of findings. Context makes sense of findings, and its loss potentially threatens to derail the synthetic project. This problem must be addressed when reviews bring the same and/or similar qualitative traditions together. However, when the outputs of radically different qualitative traditions are combined, complications pertaining to this issue increase and, also, new questions arise. Thus, mindful of Thorne's (2017) negative remarks regarding the quality of qualitative meta-synthesis (above), since researcher assumptions and ways of working differ between traditions, and these differences influence what is found as well as how findings are interpreted, extremely sophisticated methods will be needed when, for example, the findings of a Heideggerian informed phenomenological study are reviewed alongside those from a traditional field ethnography. Reviewers who tackle these sorts of problem must stay alert to the complications that integration generates, and to protect themselves from criticism, they need to be clear about the grounds on which 'a' method of synthesis is chosen.

As per Chapter 1, despite the primacy of the standard model, most methodologists list contrasting synthetic approaches. Many of these approaches reproduce essential features of the standard model. Yet they also differ from each other in subtle and sometimes not so subtle ways. Given this, reviewers who wish to tie their work to anything but the standard model must choose between approaches. On occasion, clear and straightforward reasons can be cited to support whatever choice is made and no problems exist. However, life is rarely straightforward, and if choices are to be anything other than random and arbitrary, reviewers need reasons for the decisions they take. Methodologists provide reviewers with two types of reason for their choice of synthetic approach. First, it might be asserted that a method is effective for a specific purpose. Second, philosophic and theoretical supports are given.

Effectiveness, theoretic justification, and warrant

Students and researchers who turn to methodological texts probably assume all included methods of synthesis are effective. After all, if a method is ineffective, why describe it? Yet, for the sake of argument, if we grant that all reviewers are similarly skilled (which they are not) and every method is effective (which is improbable), it remains to be proven – and it is unlikely that – all methods are equally effective. That is, just as individual qualitative studies presumably vary in quality, methods of synthesis doubtless differ in effectiveness.

Reviewers clearly want to use methods that are more rather than less effective. However, while methodologists state that this or that approach is best suited to this or that type of review, it is not clear, as previously noted, what references to effectiveness (i.e. being 'best suited' or 'most appropriate') convey. Levels or degrees of review effectiveness cannot be objectively determined. And while the term 'objective' might be protested (its use could be thought to impose overly severe criteria in assessment), no commonly agreed means exist that would allow relative effectiveness to be established. Therefore, absent objective and/or normative consensus on measurement, we cannot say 'this' rather than 'that' form of synthesis should be used. Committed proponents will claim their method is superior in some way to alternatives. Yet this is mere assertion. We can therefore park effectiveness as a useful guide. Some methods of synthesis must outperform others in various ways. However, we have no means of determining such difference, and without this ability claims regarding effectiveness are meaningless. Instead we ask, can theoretic justification provide the reasons reviewers need to justify method choices?

In describing the various choices that are on offer for pooling qualitative results, Aveyard, Payne and Preston (2016) state that Hannes and Lockwood (2011) ground meta-aggregation ("the qualitative equivalent to a meta-analysis", p. 24) on John Dewey pragmatism. This is a bold claim. Aveyard, Payne and Preston (2016) here propose that a quantitative and highly generalisable method of analysis is comparable or equivalent in importance to a form of qualitative aggregation. They also assert that a philosophic idea (one version of pragmatism) directs or underpins a review method (meta-aggregation). We may want to dispute or at least question claims regarding equivalence (considerable additional argument is required before this can be accepted). However, regards reference to Dewey, no further details are given and, thus, we might ask – when this type of assertion is made, do reviewers need to understand anything about the nature of the underpinning presented? Or, as in this instance, is it enough simply to cite a philosopher's name?

Essentially, what does offering a philosophic or theoretic justification for method choice involve and require? Note, I am not suggesting Dewey's ideas do not warrant or underpin meta-aggregation (I suspect they do not, however, for argument's sake we can accept the claim as correct), and Karin Hannes and Craig Lockwood are both respected and noted scholars (I am not criticising them or their argument). I am instead proposing that whatever this warrant amounts to remains unexplained by Aveyard, Payne and Preston (2016) and, indeed, similar justifications made by other methodologists can be equally curt. Further, across the 'how to' methodological genre, when it comes to describing the theoretic basis on which proposed methods of synthesis rest, description is often ill-defined, weak, or absent.

By providing an underpinning rationale or justification for the method advanced (i.e. in referencing Dewey), Aveyard, Payne and Preston (2016) tacitly accept the need for just this underpinning. However, no consensus on the form, depth and/or robustness of proffered theoretic justification exists. Some scholars (e.g. Booth, Papaioannou and Sutton, 2012) offer a reasonable degree of support. Others do not. And just as effectiveness is an unhelpful concept in assessing forms of synthesis (without a measure of effectiveness, claims to effectiveness and/or comparative effectiveness lack meaning), absent agreement on what counts as philosophic or theoretic warrant, it is difficult to know what type of 'warranting' information is required and, also, when enough information is provided (i.e. enough information to support the idea of warrant). Thus, while many methods of synthesis are advanced without reference to philosophic and theoretic support, even when this backing is offered, it is unclear what 'enough' and 'sufficient' support looks like in this context.

Reviewers who rely on the information contained in methodological texts will probably be confused (see Chapter 3). That is, reviewers who do not possess advanced theoretic understandings (background knowledge capable of untangling what is said), and reviewers who have not already 'taken up' a theoretic position or stance in relation to synthesis, are likely to be confounded if not mystified by the statements and explanations offered in the majority of methodological texts they encounter. Further, reviewers who wish to use philosophic and theoretic justifications to differentiate and choose between methods are unlikely to find the information provided useful. Some supporting rationales are more developed than others. However, there is no agreed means of choosing between contrasting rationales and this is a problem for reviewers anxious to justify their decisions.

On the other hand, from the perspective of a methodologist, it might be objected that 'how to' guides simply lack the space to explore these issues in depth. Thus, philosophic and theoretic justifications aplenty exist, but there may not be room to include them within the page limits available and, hence, oblique reference to justifications are all that can be included. This may be the difficulty faced by Aveyard, Payne and Preston (2016). Alternatively, the readers of methodological texts might not want to become bogged down or lost in abstract philosophic and theoretic debate. That is, action orientated reviewers (researchers and students) primarily or simply need to know what to do. And why they do what they do may be seen as less vital.

Conversely, when reviewers choose between methods of syntheses in the absence of robust explanation or understanding of the underpinnings of review options, they are, to use the vernacular, flying blind. Without this understanding, reviewers might as well roll dice to decide which approach they take, and dropping a philosopher's name into argument, even a famous one, scarcely counts as explanation. It hardly counts as anything. For example, appeals to, in this instance, pragmatic justification of the sort made by Hannes and Lockwood (2011) require unpacking.

Philosophic pragmatism, we should briefly note, is not one thing. Its adherents disagree on how the descriptor should be interpreted (Joas, 1993), and invoking the concept does not, in itself, dissolve the need for careful analysis (Bernstein, 2010). Used colloquially, pragmatism means something like 'expedient' or 'sensible' (i.e. politically feasible and/or subjectively acceptable). However, by associating or grounding claims to meta-aggregation on Dewey – Hannes and Lockwood (2011) accept that practical usefulness is the measure against which the meaning of thoughts and ideas (viz, emergent themes) are to be judged. But this is question begging. How is practical usefulness to be gauged? Rescher (2000), who comes at the issue from a pragmatic realist perspective, ties the evaluation of practical usefulness to "*matters of prediction and control*" (p. 96 – italicisation in original). This makes sense. It is at least plausible. Yet, prediction and control are strange words to link with qualitative research and this is probably not what Hannes and Lockwood (2011), or Aveyard, Payne and Preston (2016) meant to imply.

Reviewers who use a method of synthesis but have no real understanding of the grounds on which that method stands do not, in my opinion, comprehend key features of that method. If all methods were equivalently effective and supported this would not matter (perhaps). However, neither of these suppositions is likely to apply and, therefore, ignorance (i.e. not understanding) matters. Theoretic disagreement concerning the grounds on which study findings are combined is apparent across different forms of syntheses. And while a range of philosophic justificatory reasons or rationales are given to support different types of qualitative, quantitative and mixed syntheses, the positions and arguments advanced often lack coherence. The strong concept of incommensurability need not be invoked. However, justificatory criteria differ between forms of review, and contrasting justifications can be at odds. Bayesian meta-analysis, for example, uses qualitative data to develop probability distributions which are thereafter tested quantitatively (Booth, Papaioannou and Sutton, 2012, p. 157), and the assumptions operative here are clearly not those used in descriptive narrative synthesis, or the form of meta-aggregation associated with Hannes and Lockwood (2011). Reviewers choosing between approaches presumably want to understand these sorts of differences at a theoretic level. Yet how this is to be done remains unclear.

Nursing methodologists, for whatever reason, are unwilling to engage with this issue. However, where background assumptions (theories and philosophies) differ, it is not unreasonable to assume that some are more defendable (intelligible) than others. Further, within nursing's broader literature, science and evidence more generally lack agreed definitions (Thomas, 2016; Aimee, 2017; Tapp and Mireille, 2017). And, thus, disagreement on the theoretic and philosophic basis of review syntheses, and an absence of consensus on what science and evidence allow, muddy vital elements within review processes. Done well, syntheses of all sorts can generate compelling findings. Yet non-expert reviewers (i.e. most of us) are likely to need considerably more detail and information than is contained in methodological texts before anything other than simple forms of synthesis (the standard model) can realistically be attempted. Supporting rationales for these procedures are often inadequately described. The problem of divergent and conflicting rationales is underexplored, and when these problems are set alongside requirements that reviews answer questions, and that practice recommendations follow on from the resolution of these questions, it is hardly surprising that comparatively few nurses attempt or successfully master complex qualitative reviews.

Qualitative research and active citation

Chapter 6 introduced big data to illustrate the way in which changes occurring mostly outside of nursing impact on and further complicate quantitative review processes. Here active citation plays a similar role.

> The qualitative research tradition will be well served by augmenting existing citation practices with a more deliberate approach to the presentation and discussion of data. Active citation makes research more transparent and facilitates its substantiation – by making it easier for authors to show, and readers to see, the evidence on which authors

rely, and how they rely on it. Hence, the method increases … [researcher] ability to demonstrate the rigor and validity of their work, as well as to enhance its descriptive richness and interpretive depth.

(A Guide to Active Citation, 2013, p. 2)

Active citation is most developed in political science (Dafoe, 2014; Issac, 2015; Hall, 2016; Schwartz-Shea and Yanow, 2016; Johnson et al., 2017; Shesterinina, Pollack and Arriola, 2019), and while the concept summates an assortment of practices, and is used in pursuance of varied goals (e.g. impact assessment – Cai et al., 2019); at root the descriptor captures a very simple idea. Thus, researchers seek to convince readers (reviewers) that their interpretations are correct or, if that term is problematic, defendable. Journal publications do not, however, provide enough 'space' for researchers to be as informative and transparent as they want or need to be (Gaikwad, Herrera and Mickey, 2019). That is, even journals permitting long-form publications necessarily place limits on what is presented. New technology, including online or cloud based bulk data repositories, overcome this problem (see e.g. Elman, Kapiszewski and Vinuela, 2010; Karcher, Kirilova and Weber, 2016). Specifically, links or directions (sign posts) can be inserted into papers, and should readers wish to know more about a study, if readers want to see the researcher's 'workings out' (so to speak), then clicking through to this additional material dissolves publication restrictions. Active citation allows researchers to release anonymised interview transcripts and audio and other data recordings. Coding details and versions of coding (including 'false starts') can be explained in all their resplendent minutiae, and supplementary and supporting texts ('back up' material) can be provided.

Active citation is not new. However, while by 2012 the American Political Science Association Council had formalised policies guiding data access and research transparency and, variously described, active citation had evolved to become encouraged good practice (Lupia and Elman, 2014) – I am unable to locate (at the time of writing) any papers within CINAHL that discuss or make use of active citation. That said, the importance of these developments for nursing is difficult to assess. It is always conceivable that a certain amount of hype surrounds the latest trend (Synder, 2014). Nonetheless, while (as has been argued) it may be that no amount of detail and documentation can fully explain or justify the deliberations of qualitative researchers to reviewers, active citation clearly moves as far towards openness as it is possible to go and this, I suggest, can only be a good thing.

> [T]he rejection of reliability and validity in qualitative inquiry in the 1980s has resulted in an interesting shift for "ensuring rigor" from the investigator's actions during the course of the research, to the reader or consumer of qualitative inquiry. The emphasis on strategies that are implemented during the research process has been replaced by strategies for evaluating trustworthiness and utility that are implemented once a study is completed … reliability and validity remain appropriate concepts for attaining rigor in qualitative research … [and] qualitative researchers should reclaim responsibility for reliability and validity by implementing verification strategies integral and self-correcting during the conduct of inquiry itself. This ensures the attainment of rigor using strategies inherent within each qualitative design, and moves the responsibility for incorporating and maintaining reliability and validity from external reviewers' judgements to the investigators themselves.

(Morse, Barrett and Mayan, 2002, p. 13)

Morse, Barrett and Mayan (2002) note that active citation pushes responsibility for demonstrating research robustness back onto researchers, and kindred arguments are made by Moravcsik in relation to qualitative replicability, transparency and trust (2010; 2014a; 2014b). It might at this point be objected that, for example, replicability is a term associated with quantitative rather than qualitative study. However, first, as Hannes (2017) notes, some qualitative reviewers do invoke criteria linked to quantitative research in appraisal and, second, given that "there is no consensus for assessing any piece of qualitative research" (Leung, 2015, p. 325), we have no reason (bar caprice) to dismiss an interest in replicability. Moreover, third, the objection rests, I propose, on distinctions that are naïve or disputable when the aims and ambitions of those pushing for active citation are recognized. That is, within the writing of political scientists and others, we find an earnest and ongoing attempt to think through and meet the problems that qualitative inquiry is renowned for, and in this process, distinctions identified by Hannes (2017) are creatively reconfigured.

Just as big data poses a problem for nurse reviewers by highlighting and exacerbating known problems with statistical competence and comprehension – active citation or transparent reporting pushes to the forefront questions that qualitative appraisers might prefer to downplay. Thus, while nurse reviewers are or should be aware of the way in which publication norms restrict the amount of detail and explanation that researchers are permitted to provide, the existence of what appear to be superior reporting practices challenge us all to require higher standards in the reviews we conduct. This challenge will become increasingly difficult to ignore if active citation becomes better known, and to the extent that scholars outside of nursing are developing methods and forms of analysis that 'we' remain unaware of, nursing and those we care for may be ill served.

Concluding thoughts – literature or literatures?

As per Chapter 6, no attempt has been made to unpack all the issues that might potentially influence qualitative appraisal. I have not, therefore, discussed triangulation, saturation, or member checking, ideas that – along with emergence – are critiqued by Varpio et al. (2017), and others (van Rijnsoever, 2016; Saunders et al., 2018). Nor have I explored the mismatch that occasionally exists between stated qualitative theory (the principles upon which a study is purportedly grounded) and actual research practice (Lau and Traulsen, 2017), or the benefits that might accompany the big datafication of qualitative research (Latzko-Toth, Bonneau and Millette, 2017). One of my favourite bugbears, the willingness of qualitative researchers to undertake interviews and code transcripts without attempting formalised training has likewise not been explored despite good evidence that, particularly when handling sensitive subjects and/or interacting with vulnerable people, training provides tangible benefits (Powell and Wright, 2008; Goodell, Stage and Cooke, 2016). I have instead stuck with familiar themes (e.g. lack of conceptual clarity). However, to conclude, I will make one final point. Specifically, I want to note that, while reviewers refer to 'the literature', it may be more sensible to think about literatures and, if this is allowed, some of the problems identified in relation to qualitative study might be reframed.

While from the perspective of busy and harassed clinicians, students and researchers, philosophy can seem dry, abstract and irrelevant – modern work in the philosophy of science should be of interest to anyone undertaking a literature review. Scholars working within this discipline are positioning science as a plural or pluralistic rather than a unitary or unified endeavour (see e.g. Bluhm, 2014; 2017), and pluralism demands that we think about literatures rather than 'a' or 'the' literature. This is important because, among much else, it undercuts exhortations to the effect that all science must be value free and, therefore, while being value free is sometimes a laudable objective, it need not always be. Thus, although we would not expect the subjective preferences and values of researchers working on quarks to intrude into the research process (or a review of that literature), the same cannot be said of those whose work explores, for example, social justice, the meaning of compassion, or the nature of care (see Chapter 4). Potentially, pluralism opens up new ways of conceptualising the location and appraisal of diverse materials. Yet, insofar as these ideas are largely ignored within nursing, writing and thinking remains stubbornly and uncritically wedded to unitary and perhaps unhelpful conceptions of science. Earlier I suggested that a few of the components of qualitative reports look more like humanities than traditional scientific products and, maybe, this reveals or points towards an important facet of qualitative endeavour. Namely, the type of questions asked by qualitative researchers, and the methods used to address those questions are non-scientific insofar as (Chapter 2) they are not amendable to resolution in the way that quantitative and/or treatment option questions can be. It is conceivable that at least some qualitative studies should be seen as humanities products through and through; and if this is the case, alternative ways of reviewing and making sense of them – and the literatures they reference or are associated with – should be considered.

Notes

1 See Preface regards difficulties in comprehending thought processes, particularly concerning reasons (i.e. the reasons researchers offer in respect to meaning attribution).
2 This element of the critique collapses if or when qualitative work is presented in long form (e.g. monographs or similar). However, as Chapter 5 discussed, the standard model pushes nurses to look at short research reports rather than books and (Chapter 1) reading is not always valued by those conducting reviews.

8

THE FINAL CURTAIN

- Reviews do not always need to 'answer' questions in the sense normally associated with that word.
- Contemplation can validate and direct reviews.
- Humanity and arts texts should play a bigger part in many if not all reviews undertaken by nurses.
- The place and role of interest-values in communication and argument is revisited.
- Calls for wider reading and the inclusion of humanity and arts texts in reviews performed by nurses are associated with reviewer interest-values.

Although this book has only grazed the surface of a huge and complex topic, a great deal of ground has nonetheless been covered. Chapters 1 through to 5 identified key review activities and concepts that require clarification. Specifically, the phrasing of a review's purpose, question, and scope are not always clearly enunciated and, potentially, this obfuscates or confuses review processes. Further, crucial terms such as 'comprehensive range' and 'relevant' are attached to 'evidence' without settled understanding accompanying their usage and, again, this is unhelpful. To give life to the arguments presented, a 'good' search was described. It was suggested that had this search been performed differently, 'better' or more informative sources would have been located. (The use of scare quotes hints at the difficulties encountered in defining these terms.) It was also proposed that non-nursing and non-research texts could and possibly should have been accessed. Aspects of the evaluation of quantitative and qualitative research were then described and it was asserted that non-expert reviewers face considerable hurdles in evaluating these forms of evidence. Thus, underprepared nurses may fail to establish that quantitative statistical tests are correctly chosen and run and, should this occur, the assessment of results is undercut and appraisal remains incomplete. Alternatively, absent agreement on what constitutes a good qualitative report, reviewers are challenged in principle to determine both the trustworthiness of findings and appropriate (defendable) forms of synthesis. Developments outside of nursing that complicate the review of quantitative and qualitative sources were identified and – to restress comments made previously – the arguments presented in this book are neither anti-research or anti-scientific.

Professional ambition

Across the work common sets of assumptions and practices that are taught to and used by possibly the majority of nurse reviewers have been problematised. Labelled the standard model, these methods have merit and their use is frequently appropriate. That said, it has been argued that reviewers may not always need to answer questions in the manner pre-scribed by this model. The use of humanity and arts texts was promoted, and it was proposed that reviewers who recognise the role played by personal interests and values in the review process might endow those interests-values with a constructive function. As should be apparent, these arguments presume a notion of professional identity and ambition that stands apart from that espoused by at least some nurses.

How nurses think about and approach searches and reviews has repeatedly been tied to constructions of professional identity. At the extreme, it is suggested that concepts of pro-fessionalism which valorise the establishment and maintenance of strict disciplinary boundaries potentially compromise the feasibility of learning from non-nursing literatures and allied workers (see Preface and Chapter 1). However, less excitedly, criticisms contained in this book – criticisms focused on the questionable methodological robustness of some review practices – challenge ambition more generally. That is, while professionalising rhetoric talks up notions of excellence and best practice, many nurses (students, educators, researchers) seem willing to overlook problems that threaten the coherence and rationality of review processes.

On the other hand, despite the sombre catalogue of woes outlined in preceding chapters, excellent reviews are conducted; and journals such as *Nursing Ethics, Nursing Inquiry* and *Nursing Philosophy* regularly publish papers that – if not reviews – evidence the type of wide reading and meaningful analysis that is advocated for in this book. This suggests elements of what is argued for already occur and, at root, this work merely proposes that, vis-à-vis reviews, narrow approaches to reading should be discouraged and additional methodological development is required. These are modest suggestions, and whilst their acceptance throws out complex questions, as emphasised, not only do most methodologists cite alternatives to the standard model (the primary focus of opprobrium), they also sketch strategies offering useful guidance to students, researchers and clinicians.

Further, although the claim that nurse reviewers must address and seek to answer specific questions in every instance has been poo-pooed, this way of proceeding is, of course, often perfectly sensible. Arguing that something need not be attempted in all cases is not to say it need never be attempted. And the idea that non-answerable (non-resolvable) questions rela-ted to theoretic and normative/evaluative topics can be suitable objects for review is not antithetical to a focus on answerable questions when appropriate. Indeed, addressing answerable questions may be laudable in the vast majority of instances albeit that, vis-à-vis evidence-based healthcare, literatures from "the social sciences (e.g. sociology, social psy-chology, anthropology) and humanities (e.g. philosophy, literature/storytelling, design) … [inevitably complement or underpin the] intellectual basis" of this activity (Greenhalgh, 2018, p. 1). And, thus, even when clinically grounded and answerable (scientific) questions are asked, cross-disciplinary and non-research texts might and frequently should be sourced by reviewers when the 'basis' of activity is considered.

A tentative conclusion

That reviewers may, in some circumstances, seek out sources that cannot resolve questions in the manner prescribed by the standard model can be tied to the idea that contemplation is a good in and of itself. Reviewers who permit this possibility might turn to the literature simply to explore (with more or less degrees of structure) what is known or believed about a subject or subject field. And while contemplation may result in action (i.e. practice change), reviews undertaken in this way need not begin with or develop formal or answerable questions. To further this idea 'attention' is introduced as a possibly useful concept in envisioning reviews. Hannah Arendt's writing on contemplation is thereafter presented and, following this, examples of the potential use value of humanity and arts texts in reviews are provided. To conclude the chapter, the place of interests-values in reviews is again revisited. However, prior to this, two points deserve consideration.

First, arguments in this final section of the book are unavoidably tentative. Positively, in the 'real world', I have observed colleagues reading in ways that suggest they are in fact undertaking quite sophisticated reviews merely because subjects or lines of inquiry interest them – and researchers and clinicians occasionally also do this thing (caveats concerning time and resources notwithstanding). In these instances, reading, thinking and discussion might be described as contemplative or exploratory. These self-directed reviews (assuming the descriptor applies) do not seek to resolve questions in the instrumental means–ends manner presumed by the standard model. Contemplative or curiosity driven reviews are thus undertaken and, crucially, they have value for those engaging in them. However, that said, it must be acknowledged that where professionals read to inform practice, removing requirements around question setting, and degrading the necessity that change should be an anticipated goal, is not without problem. Contemplation can be considered self-indulgent. It is unlikely to attract funding or institutional support (see Petrovskaya, McDonald and McIntyre, 2011), and it runs counter to the antipathy to reading that was recognised in Chapter 1.

Second, while accepting the legitimacy of contemplative reviews significantly increases the case for humanity and arts texts being designated 'relevant' location objects, the inclusion of these sources in reviews does not rely on the idea of contemplation. That is, claims favouring the inclusion of humanity and arts texts do not rest on accepting the cogency of contemplation as a method or type of review. Nonetheless, contemplation and wide reading of the sort promoted here are mutually supportive or complementary.

Attention

If reviews are undertaken so that reviewers can learn from the literature (broadly defined), it might also be allowed that what is read (located and appraised) sustains learning in relation to 'attention'. Two versions of attention are identified.

First, reviewer attention is *required* or demanded by relevant texts whose internal logic appears plausible. Scientific reports demonstrate plausibility or warrant (trustworthiness) when they describe the use of methods and tools that are truth conducive (valid and reliable). That is, methods and tools that produce or identify evidence. However, non-research scholarship also establishes the plausibility of its claims (conclusions) when the grounds (premises) on which those claims are made are carried in argument. Non-research papers may therefore petition reviewer attention on essentially the same reliabilist grounds that research reports do.

That is, scholarship can, when the rationality of argument is granted, when conclusions appear defensible, require reviewer attention (i.e. in relation to the object of interest, what is said cannot reasonably be ignored).

Alternatively, second, attention is *grabbed* when interest proves directive. Thus, irrespective of the logic or plausibility of argument, attention is seized when an idea – deemed relevant – is presented to or imagined by the reviewer on the basis of what is read. In Chapter 5 it was asserted that, for me, a text by Guggenbühl-Craig (2015) provided or stimulated ideas which, in relation to the object of review, were considered pertinent. In this instance, although I was persuaded by what was argued, persuasion rested on my willingness or disposition to accept and 'make something' of what was read. That is, some aspect of what was said – something other or in addition to logic/evidence – compelled me to connect (coherentism) what I took to be proposed with the subject under review.

Logic and/or evidence can be tested and attention in the first *required* sense lends itself to public scrutiny. Interest, on the other hand, is subjectively *grabbed* and imagined rather than demonstrated. Nevertheless, regardless of how attention is gained, what is learnt or realised ought, arguably, to inform review processes. This informing may facilitate or allow a question to be answered. However, it need not necessarily do so. Reviewers might become better informed and/or more insightful about subjects without setting or concluding questions and, clearly, the directive and interpretive importance of reviewer concerns and the values underpinning them re-emerge when attention is considered.

Contemplation

It may not be necessary to support the idea that contemplation is a good in and of itself. The idea is so self-evidently sensible that, in many respects, it simply 'stands'. Further, if this is the case, perhaps we can allow that, with the addition of a few additional premises, contemplation might represent or be a viable or legitimate review method or methodology. Alternatively, if contemplation needs support, a varied list of names can be recruited for this purpose. Here the writing of Hannah Arendt (1906–1975),[1] is enlisted to carry a version of contemplation. However, Aristotle (2009) would equally suffice.

In *The Human Condition* (1998), Arendt sets out a 'just so' story. The historical narrative presented might be challenged. Nonetheless, like Hobbe's man in a state of nature, Rousseau's social contract, or Rawl's original position – Arendt suggests ideas that are of interest even if the precise details of what is described are of questionable accuracy. Thus, in synopsis, it is proposed that activity can be classified in three ways. 'Labour' describes activities that are consumed or used up in their production (e.g. washing or toileting another person). Labour thus envisaged is contrasted with or against work as 'craft'. That is, making things which outlive their immediate use (e.g. documenting a care plan). Further, alongside labour and craft, Arendt describes 'action'. Action takes place in the social or public realm. It includes those things we think of as politics (widely defined) and also, peculiarly, thoughtful contemplation. For Arendt, these activities exist within a hierarchy. Historically, the contemplative life outranked political life, which outranked craft work, which outranked labour. However, in the modern era – and her story spans millennia – labour has become exalted, contemplation is diminished, and insofar as it lacks instrumental use value, contemplation is despised.

Between Past and Future (2006) explores the notion that use value and contemplation are at odds. Here it is noted that in Plato's "parable of the cave, the philosopher leaves the cave in search of the true essence of Being without a second thought to the practical applicability of what he is going to find" (Arendt, 2006, p. 112). This is significant. The insight allows that, while practical applicability may derive from contemplation, beneficial gains are not expected. Instead they are merely a pleasant if unsort side effect and, thus, Arendt disaggregates thinking as contemplation from reasoning aimed at the production of truth/knowledge. Conceptualised in this way, contemplation is its own reward or endpoint, and contra the sort of means/ends calculation that supposedly structures modern discourse:

> To expect truth to come from thinking signifies that we mistake the need to think with the urge to know. Thinking can and must be employed in the attempt to know, but in the exercise of this function it is never itself; it is the handmaiden of an altogether different exercise.
>
> *(Arendt, 1971, p. 61)*

Ramming this point home, and to emphasise that thinking cannot be reduced to problem solving, Arendt placed the following quotation from Heidegger's *What Is Called Thinking?* (1976 [1954]) at the beginning of the introduction to her *The Life of the Mind* (1971)[2]:

> Thinking does not bring knowledge as do the sciences.
> Thinking does not produce usable practical wisdom.
> Thinking does not solve the riddles of the universe.
> Thinking does not endow us directly with the power to act.
>
> *(Arendt, 1971, p. 1)*

This is strong meat – and the argument it supports enables Arendt to establish contemplation as the search for meaning (a search that never ends), through the posing of unanswerable questions. This conception of contemplation differs dramatically from the idea that thinking aims, solely, at settling truth or knowledge claims (i.e. closing questions). Yet, at the same time, contemplation scaffolds truth and knowledge for, if mankind forgets to ask unanswerable questions, if contemplation is abandoned, our ability to resolve that which is answerable is endangered.

> [D]rawing a distinguishing line between truth and meaning … I do not wish to deny that thinking's quest for meaning and knowledge's quest for truth are connected.… It is more [that] … men, if they were ever to lose the appetite for meaning we call thinking and cease to ask unanswerable questions, would lose … the capacity to ask all the answerable questions.
>
> *(Arendt, 1971, pp. 61–62)*

Contemplation's value does not then derive from its ability to answer or close questions. Rather, contemplation allows us to better reflect on and understand that which refuses closure. Contemplation or thinking can resolve puzzles. Indeed, the types of answerable question prized by those following the standard model cannot be settled in contemplation or thinking's absence. However, contemplation facilitates more than this and, I suggest, when anything other than technical and/or the simplest of treatment option problems interest reviewers, Arendt's idea of contemplation is worth considering since, possibly, it holds out a means of articulating and thereby defending an approach to reviewing that standard model procedural guides cannot match.

Significantly, for Arendt, contemplation involves both a "deliberate act of abstaining" (ibid., p. 93), and "looking upon something from the outside" (ibid., p. 93). It positions the contemplator as a spectator rather than an actor, and while this facilitates understanding, understanding in this sense demands a "withdrawal from doing" (ibid., p. 93). That is, critical thought requires a turning away from blind partisanship.[3] This does not, however, make contemplation passive or politically quietist. Arendt was no such person. Values overtly structured her thought and deeds, and while contemplators 'stand back', contemplation is, ultimately, supremely active. Put simply, we contemplate or think about, as well as with, others. And, for reviewers, that is, people whose endeavours encompass or centre on the type of thoughtful engagement with the claims of others that Arendt's description of contemplation engages, these ideas provide, in my view, a method or methodology which, depending upon the type of question asked, may – ironically – be of use.

Humanities and arts texts in reviews

Like her friend Camus and onetime lover Heidegger, Arendt's style of exposition defies easy deconstruction. Her writing is logical (propositional statements are advanced). However, the manner in which she weaves together intricate social, political, historical and psychological themes means the resulting analysis is layered and complex. (I am thus painfully aware of the inadequacy of my brief description – above – of her conception of contemplation.) Positively, Arendt's form of expression enables much to be 'unfolded' or made accessible that might otherwise remain hidden. Nevertheless, unfortunately, for those who favour Manichean arguments and positions of the black and white variety, Arendt will disappoint. Therefore, to avoid becoming bogged down in constant references back to this or that interpretation of Arendt, the idea that contemplation or the contemplative way is or might be of service to reviewers is henceforth pursued through the claim, oft repeated, that humanity and arts scholarship has a potential role to play in reviews. The background assumption here is that these sorts of text can be recognised and 'deployed' by reviewers who adopt something like Arendt's position (although, as previously stated, this adoption is not strictly necessary for their value to be realised).

Student number one

Guggenbühl-Craig's book *Power in the Helping Professions* (2015) was introduced in Chapter 5 as an example problem for those following standard model precepts. Specifically, it was asked: how or in what way (if at all) could this sort of non–nursing and non-standard research text be included in reviews performed by nurses? Here, mindful of the legitimacy of contemplation as a review 'methodology', two new non-research texts are described. It is proposed that, again, in context, it is possible to argue that each is 'relevant'. That is, they might both find a place in reviews.

Thus, I recently supervised the Independent Studies (dissertations) of two students both of whom focused on aspects of end-of-life and terminal care. The first student explored aspects of bereavement support. She was concerned about the emotional impact of death on survivors and her work examined how, before and after death, relatives and friends could be 'prepared' and subsequently helped. In what is titled the discussion section of the study this student noted, briefly, that while nurses seek to reduce the trauma associated with bereavement among survivors, there is something about the 'sadness' of death which, perhaps, ought to be 'held on to'. In short, when supporting bereaved relatives/friends, nurses might need to respect and cherish as well as assuage negative emotional experiences.

This normatively charged idea was discussed during support meetings but, bar passing reference, it was expunged from submitted work. Insofar as the student was interested in evaluative or normative aspects of the idea, since healthcare databases may not be the best place to locate texts dealing with evaluative/normative concepts, and given my institution's preference for the standard model of literature review formatting, this was probably sensible. However, it is also somewhat deflating. Problematically, as described, research in its traditional guise addresses questions about what 'is' (answerable questions) rather than what 'ought' to be (unanswerable questions), and because the student's insight pointed towards the type of judgements that empiric investigation cannot or cannot easily resolve, dropping this line of inquiry protected the student from entering what, from the perspective of the standard model, is a difficult space. On the other hand, the student had encroached upon a fascinating and possibly important subject (an element or dimension of bereavement experience/care that is not perhaps adequately recognised), and had the literature review been structured differently – if non-standard review model approaches were promoted, allowed or sought out – humanity and arts texts might have been recruited which, definitional problems notwithstanding, could have engaged this issue in ways that may be considered 'relevant' and 'helpful'.

For example, Aldous Huxley's dystopian novel *Brave New World* (2007, [1932]) includes the 'death ward' scene (Chapter 14) in which John, one of the principle characters, visits his dying mother (Linda). John is incensed by the cheery way death is actualised, and he is repulsed by the manner in which (Delta) children are encultured not to fear death by playing between the beds of the dying. In the world of the novel these are clearly, from John's perspective, 'bads'. However, arguably, if nurses could intervene to abolish the often-harrowing emotional distress that accompanies death, this might be considered a 'good'. Linda certainly does not object to what is happening (she is enveloped in Soma/drug induced bliss) and, if feasible, Huxley's 'nightmare' of desensitisation would lessen some if not all of the trauma associated with bereavement. The ease with which this goal is accomplished in the novel is implausible. Nonetheless, the objective chased is comprehendible. It has merit. And, yet, *Brave New World* cleverly captures something about the sacrosanct or vital significance of death that would be lost if, by whatever means, its sting was pulled. To some extent then this text pursues a point addressed by the student's concern/insight. But, in a review performed by a nurse, a review conducted to inform thinking about practice, can arts products such as this legitimately inform what is produced or concluded?

> [I]magination is necessary, not only to art but also to knowledge. It essentially provides unity to the multitude of impressions that our senses present us with. It does this through an act that both synthesizes and schematizes.
>
> *(Swedberg, 2014, p. 192)*

Swedberg (2014) here references Kant, and Kant's influence on Arendt. It is suggested that imaginative insight collates and structures what is realised and, in this way, imagination informs thinking. Indeed, in some contexts imagination and thinking might be considered synonyms. Further, even though its influence remains underdescribed, imagination is as crucial in research as it is in the arts or humanities. Its remit cannot be bounded (Jung, 2001 [1933]). That said, imagination clearly dominates arts products, and the relation between imagination and truth/knowledge is complex. Bullishly, Tanney (2013) ties fictive imagination to knowledge when she claims that, should the concept of pride be inspected, "you'd want to read *Pride and Prejudice* … that's a lovely study on the notion of pride", and Stock (2016) likewise argues that fiction can, potentially, generate understanding, knowledge and self-truth. Camus (2013 [1951]) is even more declamatory. He proposes (in a discussion on Proust) that "the novel can reconstruct creation itself" (ibid., p. 211), and potentially at least, artistic reconstruction transfigures and regenerates all that is true and/or truly matters.

The role that texts such as *Brave New World* (2007) might play in grounding knowledge/understanding is, therefore, widely accepted. Yet, problematically, while Huxley is a respected and acclaimed author, we are here referencing 'merely' a novel. Works of fiction are not usually seen as sources of evidence. They do not have a place in the standard model, and many nurses will undoubtedly be uncomfortable with the idea that this or kindred texts could appear or be quoted in the reviews they undertake.

> In a work of imaginative fiction, Huxley (2007) suggests that death's negative emotional impact potentially has worth or value. The role of perspective is recognised to be important in this valuing and, significantly, the full nature and form of what is proposed remains underdetermined. Nonetheless, if Huxley's (ibid.) insight is granted, it might be argued that – in caring for those who are dying and, also, bereaved family and friends – nurses should remain alert to the beneficial (albeit unbidden) possibilities that attend otherwise painful emotional experience. This idea is relevant to this review because …

I also harbour qualms and, thus, brashly asserting that "Death's negative emotional impact potentially has worth or value (Huxley, ibid.)" would, on its own, probably push the use of arts sources in reviews too far (the claim is overly strident). However, the more caveated statement (above) is one I could accept.

To be carried, this sort of claim may need to more comprehensively recognise the referenced narrative. That is, just as research reports explain how findings are derived in order that warrant can be established, so – where arts texts are cited in reviews – readers might require relevant passages to be reproduced so that they can judge whether the idea or claim being advanced 'holds'.[4] Alternatively, if the idea-claim presented was inspired by what was read (rather than being stated in what was read), an explanation of the logic-reasoning connecting cited sources with reviewer interpretation is presumably necessary. (However, note, this reproduces problems introduced earlier around qualitative report analysis.) Nevertheless, statements such as that made above could be acceptable if situated within or alongside subsidiary references to personal insight/experience and/or supporting or disconfirming research findings. Or, they might be placed relative to other confirmatory and/or disconfirmatory arts and humanity sources.[5] Thus, located within argument, I believe the use of arts texts in reviews can be defended and, moreover, their use is mandated (a deliberately strong term) when inclusion develops understanding in pertinent ways that are unexplored or unsanctioned in or by research findings.

Accepting or rejecting this proposal hinges on, amongst other things, whether reviews are envisaged solely as vehicles that answer questions using research evidence (take a standard model approach) or, instead, whether more contemplative constructions are permitted. In conversation with colleagues (a haphazard but productive source of ideas), it is evident that two categories of reaction are generated by the claims outlined here. Either they are rejected out of hand 'That's not acceptable', 'Absolutely not'. Or they are seen as reasonable and unremarkable 'Of course', 'No problem'. There appears to be little appetite for a middle position.

Student number two

The second student sought to explore the 'lived experience' of those dying from cancer so that she could, thereafter, hopefully better care for and support such patients. Or, rather, to pass a piece of academic work she looked at a tiny subset of research reports produced by those who claim to describe something of such experience.

While her subject could be tackled in several ways, this student searched for and tried to make sense of primarily qualitative reports (mainly phenomenological studies located via CINAHL). In this undertaking difficulties were repeatedly encountered when papers dealing with the unique experience of unrepresentative others were read with a view to drawing lessons for general use (i.e. she sought to generalise non-generalisable research findings). Moreover, the student found it hard to assess the quality of reports in the absence of consensus on what 'good' qualitative studies look like. (Both problems were discussed in Chapter 7.) Nonetheless, these issues aside, over coffee we talked about the enigmatic and mutable nature of death literatures (see e.g. Jernigan, Wadiak and Wang, 2019), and the potential of first-person narratives rather than 'distanced' non-first-person research studies to inform her work was discussed – and rejected. She was adamant that monographs would not be considered. They were 'too long'.

That said, large numbers of texts written by those who are or were themselves dying now exist, and within this literature, I greatly admire Gillian Rose's *Love's Work: A Reckoning With Life* (2011 [1995]). However, as with Huxley (2007), would it be sensible to recommend Rose (2011) to someone performing a review on the subject of the experience of dying?

While difficult to situate within genres, Rose (2011) presents, in my view, an outstanding if idiosyncratic example of a narrative dealing with death from a first-person perspective. *Love's Work* is an urgent and serious autobiography, a profoundly personal and at times disturbing memoir, a sociology, and a philosophical phenomenology on the subject of the author's then impending demise (Rose died of cancer aged 48 in 1995).[6] In her review of the book, Tubbs (1998) emphasised the role that protest plays in Rose's thinking. However, one could equally identify or highlight Rose's refusal to accept generalising tropes or ways of constructing individual experience – including individual understandings of death – and Evans (1998) conveys something of this in highlighting Rose's denial of "particular forms of knowledge" (p. 28). See also Gorman (2001) on Rose's "ethic of singularity" (p. 25).

Love's Work (2011) therefore pushes back against many of the assumptions held or made by healthcare workers regards what might be described as thanatologically correct ways of dying (i.e. 'our' interpretation of what a good death is or involves), and if I wanted to think through what death can mean, then this is a work I would turn to. Indeed, for me, Rose's book stimulates considerably more subjective insight, and it challenges taken for granted assumptions about death's meanings (plural), more effectively than any quantitative or qualitative research paper I recall. On the other hand, the work is not an easy read. The book takes time to digest and it requires, perhaps, multiple readings. Further, the book makes statements that are likely to offend, and given these 'problems', maybe students and early career researchers should avoid it?

Except, this is silly. When reviews aim to answer questions, and when arts and/or humanities scholarship can materially contribute to and nuance question resolution, these non-research sources ought to be considered. Alternatively, irrespective of settling questions, when reviews are undertaken to enhance understanding, if the purpose of the exercise is to stimulate thought, then – when non-research texts can do these things as well if not better than research reports – surely we should overtly and deliberately locate and appraise such sources? Qualitative studies, it must be remembered, sell themselves on not dissimilar grounds to those which are claimed here for humanities and arts scholarship. That is, qualitative researchers who renounce generalisation demand attention for their work on the basis that it stimulates insight and challenges and facilitates understanding. And, if these criteria ground the inclusion of qualitative material in reviews, why not Rose? Why not Huxley? Of course, introducing texts of this sort into searches is highly problematic and, as noted, concerns described in relation to qualitative analysis resurface when humanity and arts texts are considered in this way. (I have no interest in minimising the difficulties involved.) However, to repeat, 'why not'?

Cherry picking

Justifying the presence of arts and humanity texts in reviews is difficult to accommodate within or against standard model norms. That is, if this sort of material is considered 'relevant' (and I propose that, depending on context, it can or may be this thing), since these sources cannot be mechanistically identified using the databases and/or search tools most nurses are familiar with, logical or systematic grounds for establishing inclusion/exclusion are compromised, and searches that include these texts are unlikely to be able to claim they are systematic in the way this term is currently described.

Critiques regarding the objectivity and value neutrality of systematic reviews question whether the term denotes the thing it purports to do (see e.g. Castañeda, 2019). However, Aveyard, Payne and Preston (2016) highlight widely held worries about the potential of bias to distort non-systematic location strategies when they note: "The importance of a rigorous approach to reviewing the literature, rather than simply 'cherry picking' literature that is relevant to your review … is increasingly being recognised" (p. ix).[7] Aveyard, Payne and Preston (2016), and others (e.g. Goldacre, 2014a), believe this issue can be overcome through the use of a 'rigorous approach' (i.e. systematisation). Yet, first, I do not want to exclude material of the sort described above. And, second, if searcher interests and beliefs-values are granted a place in location and appraisal processes it seems implausible that unsystematically sourced materials can be excluded when they 'grab' or 'require' reviewer attention. Thus, although a demonstration of systematic search methods in the writing of reviews by students and researchers is demanded, and locating material non-systematically raises extremely knotty issues, it would be unfortunate if ostensibly sensible processes lead to relevant material – that is, relevant for or to arguments presented by reviewers – being overlooked or dismissed.

Meaningful engagement – professional ambition

Reviews undertaken by nurses regularly invoke or 'speak to' issues examined by scholars and thinkers who are not researchers. These issues might reference central topics in the sources being critiqued. Or, they may be implicated in analysis and discussion more generally. In both instances, when reviewers take up questions possessing significant economic, ethical/ normative, historical, philosophic/theoretic, policy, political or sociological aspects, they could – assuming meaningful or substantive engagement is sought – deliberately seek out and cite non-scientific and non-nursing literatures where these add to or clarify understanding. Not to do so, in my opinion, signals a peculiar lack of ambition, and to illustrate this point I here present an example from sociology.

Many nursing studies make use of sociological concepts and theories, and when appraising these reports, reviewers will want to stay alert to the way in which contrasting concepts and theories are deployed in located sources. Studies of investigations into some aspect of 'role' or 'organisational development' or, alternatively, some facet of 'change management' may, for example, conceptualise agent-structure relations in more than one way and, significantly, it is not necessarily the case that findings from reports adopting radically divergent approaches to this issue can sensibly be elided (Lipscomb, 2017a). Therefore, just as it was argued in Chapter 7 that because their grounding assumptions were at odds, some types of qualitative research are difficult to synthesise – likewise – it should not be assumed that sociological studies which accept individual and/or group agents form ('bottom up') the causal or driving force in institutional change are necessarily compatible (capable of synthesis) with reports that grant causal power to ('top down') structural forces over or against the activities of agents. In this instance, both sociologically informed papers may seemingly deal with the same subject matter. Yet the background and theoretical assumptions 'in play' underpin fundamentally divergent approaches to understanding and – because of this – simplistic comparisons may be precluded.

Reviewers aware of such issues will seek out clarificatory texts (e.g. humanities scholarship dealing with sociological theory) that describe and unravel the meaning/implications of these differences. However, reviewers who are unaware of the difficulties they confront will stumble on in ignorance and, thus, they run the risk of producing confused conclusions. Once again, this aspect of the review process remains underexplored and, self-evidently, similar arguments can be made regards the economic, ethical/normative, historical, philosophic/theoretic, policy and political claims and references contained in research reports.

Alternatively, a review following standard model presumptions might address a question along the lines of: What is the most effective pain control medication for patients with condition 'x' and comorbidities 'y' in context 'z'? In this instance quantitative research papers and systematic reviews of quantitative reports will predominantly be sourced and it may, erroneously, be imagined that non-research texts are irrelevant here. However, insofar as humanities and arts sources 'unpack' issues of value more extensively and comprehensively than empiric research generally does, and since even the most value free or value neutral of facts are interpreted and made use of in normatively charged circumstances, humanities/arts texts and the arguments and ideas they contain should not, potentially, be ignored. Indeed, even when their influence is marginal, the inclusion of humanities/arts literatures in purely 'clinical' reviews is justified when reviewers examine the (often implicit) way values and other background assumptions frame understanding (i.e. their own, as well as those built into the reports being appraised).

Values re-revisited

These comments (above) return us to the topic of values. But what are values? Various definitions exist. However, let us grant that values denote and are bestowed upon that which is preferred or scorned. Values identify "objects of desire and attitude" (Weissman, 1993, p. 3). They find expression in the core, fundamental or motivating principles by which individuals and (arguably) groups prioritise the qualities they esteem. Values ground the premises determining standards for discrimination and action. Significantly, consciously or otherwise values are formed by, influence, and often 'stand behind' belief (so values and beliefs are frequently mutually constitutive). Epistemic integrity was discussed in Chapter 4. However, advancing on what was said there, truth's relation to value, and fact-value distinctions also deserve attention. Thinking about these issues is important. Values play a crucial role in structuring argument and whatever version of reviews is favoured, this structuring facility is one reviewers ought to consider.

Values *constitute* what is taken to be true in some circumstances and *regulate* in others (Peirce, 1877; Weissman, 1993). Values are *constitutive* when, self-referentially, the methods or ways of proceeding that we use to make sense of the world are limited to or governed by interests. For example, if the authority of others is construed as being protective, and if protection is something reviewers perceive to be in their interest, reviewers could accept as correct Cochrane or CDC findings solely or predominantly on the basis of the protective authority (i.e. the legitimatisation) of authorship. Or, mindful of previous discussion of Huxley (2007) and Rose (2011), these texts are relevant for me (in the context of the study topics being explored) because I 'grasp' or recognise the values expressed in them as meeting my interests (here, an interest in the subjects being investigated). In both instances, values constitute what is true for me or us and, notably, these truths need not be true for others.

Alternatively, *regulative* principles are operative when truth separates from value in an impartial sense. By this I mean, desiring some state of affairs to exist, a review may be conducted to identify literature pertaining to the attractive or hoped for contention. Yet, if a search reveals empiric (measurable and objective) evidence refuting what we want to be the case, it would be foolish and irrational to claim that what is desired is what obtains. Clear cut instances in which this occurs may be rare. Nonetheless, a priori or established values "have referents only if there is a pre-established harmony between the world and our ideas of it or if there is direct apprehension of the things signified" (Weissman, 1993, p. 17). When regulatory truth-value conditions apply, values referencing states of affairs in the world cannot be known or claimed as true on the basis of intuition, and the confirmation of postulated truths is – comparatively – value free. Scientific hypotheses testing represents, caveats notwithstanding, a strong version of the regulatory principle.

While other 'options' exist, the constitutive-regulative distinction provides a potentially useful way into thinking about values and truth. Specifically, this schema offers a language through which the part played by values in steering comprehension can be appreciated without succumbing to the erroneous conclusion that truth is merely what value tells us it is.

Then again, reviewers might consider fact-value distinctions in argumentative structure. Cottrell (2005) describes facts as "items of information that can be checked and proved through experience, direct observation, testing and comparison" (p. 141), whereas opinions (grounded partly on values), are merely beliefs that lack "proof or substantial evidence" (p. 141). Facts in this context are objective (i.e. capable of external verification) and opinion-values are subjective (i.e. they are the products of untested and perhaps untestable rumination). At a rudimentary level statements such as "patients ought to receive healthcare on the basis of need rather than ability to pay" and "patients receive healthcare on the basis of need rather than ability to pay" are plainly different things. The first (ought) claim references a value position. The second states, in a UK context, a fact for many if not all forms of healthcare. And while values differ (not everyone favours nationalised healthcare), facts, as framed here (i.e. what 'is'), are publicly determinable.

While in academic and scientific discourse it is sometimes supposed that description should be accurate, factual, and free of value judgements – the idea that facts can be contrasted against or in opposition to values is criticised. Reviewers should remain mindful of fact-value relations. However, the idea that description can be value neutral is difficult to sustain. Thompson (2002) states that "We cannot begin to evaluate someone's reasoning if we do not understand it, or if we understand the words but fail to grasp that reasons are being offered for accepting a point of view" (p. 5). This is sensible. Yet what are reviewers to make of reasons and/or arguments that use or rely on value referents? That is, most health-related discourse.

Facts and values can often be disaggregated. Nonetheless, complication abounds where words and phrases simultaneously carry factual *and* evaluative connotations. Hare (1964) recognised that "almost every word in our language is capable of being used on occasion as a value-word (that is, for commending or its opposite)" (p. 79), and he went on to add "it is only by cross-examining a speaker that we can tell whether he is so using a word" (p. 80) (see also Wittgenstein, 1969). Factual statements can therefore be – they often are – normatively loaded, and Berlin (1998a [1953]) noted that: "Those who are concerned with human affairs are committed to the use of the moral categories and concepts" (p. 188). This statement goes on to tie commitment to 'normal' rather than scientific discourse. Nonetheless, arguably, moral and evaluative referents are implicated in both normal *and* formal or scientific language use and, however used, moral concepts and values generate meaning.

For example, a small trial into the impact of a nurse-led telephone intervention programme for patients with heart failure (Stavrianopoulos, 2016) introduced value referents to scaffold and give shape to the facts being presented. Heart failure thus "imposes a severe financial strain" on services (p. 1), and this condition "negatively" (p. 1) impacts upon the quality of life of sufferers. On the other hand, beneficially, the intervention had a "positive effect" (ibid., p. 4), and those in receipt of the service had "greatly reduced" (p. 4) hospital readmission rates. In this report, imposing a financial strain and negatively effecting quality of life are 'bads', while having a positive effect and reducing hospital readmissions are 'goods'. Value referents thus both set the scene (i.e. they identify the bads to be addressed) and they legitimise or make sense of results (where bads are overcome). Reviewers might wish to distinguish between and perhaps challenge aspects of the values wrapped up in these statements. That is, it could be argued that reducing the financial burden of care is a lesser or reduced priority compared to (despite its contested nomenclature and status) quality of life issues. Or, if 'lesser' is the wrong word, financial probity and quality of life could signify, in this instance, different kinds of value. Nonetheless, this aside, it is patently evident that values play an integral and structuring role in writing and argument. Values give meaning to facts and without this meaning enabling framework, data lacks sense and impact.

In this particular case it would be surprising if anyone objected to the value positions taken. However, contentious or potentially contentious evaluative claims and assumptions liberally litter the nursing literature and – regardless of whether they are controversial or not – reviewers need, I suggest, to comprehend when and how values enter into communication. This ability is required in order that the part taken by values in articulating and giving form to what is said can be appreciated. Yet reviewers will search in vain for substantive discussion of this topic by nursing's review methodologists.

Put another way, like scholarship, science and its products come to us in the form of argument (Kuhn, 1993; 2010), and because values infuse argument, even ostensibly strict empirical research reports rest on or incorporate moral, political and other value backed assumptions (Anderson, 2004; see also Latimer and Gómez, 2019). The influence of values on the identification and interpretation of facts-propositions and hence the contribution of values to the conclusions that are drawn usually pass, however, without acknowledgement. And in consequence, while the findings and conclusions of research and scholarship evidence the close interplay and occasional fusion of facts-propositions and opinions-values, by excluding values from consideration (analysis), reviewers may mistakenly assume that scientific results and scholarly outputs rest solely on rational criteria (where rational signals value absence or neutrality). This is almost always a mistake. It is not irrational to involve or make use of value judgements in argument. Yet since values are always or generally contestable, when their influence is cloaked, this disputable element is modulated and a false sense of certitude is generated.

Thus, in contrast to the heart failure example introduced above, imagine a reviewer interested in some aspect of healthcare organisation and financing who chances upon Hussey's (2012) discursive paper 'Just Caring'. Hussey is quite upfront about the (communitarian) value position adopted in this work, and nailing his colours to the mast he states that "it is not always clear that rights such as the freedom to choose must take precedence over equality or need" (p. 7). The paper argues for compulsory collective provision over or against voluntary or individual choice, and a range of value-soaked background assumptions and terms are woven into what is said. Hussey must be commended for his clarity. However, other writers are not always so virtuous. Oftentimes value referents are introduced covertly and/or evaluative positions are implicitly assumed. It is not always clear that authors are consciously aware of what they are doing, and the significance or role of values in argument is rarely made explicit. This creates muddle for reviewers and while, for example, Hussey's argument ought to be rejected by anyone who preferences choice over equity, this rejection requires that the part played by values in argument be understood. In this instance the position advanced is, as stated, explicit and open. Yet reviewers can come to accept 'as correct' results or conclusions that might better be described as evaluative 'interpretations'.

Interpretation

Incorporating interpretations into understanding is not necessarily problematic (in part, this is what is advocated for in relation to Huxley, 2007; Rose, 2011; and Guggenbühl-Craig, 2015). It should also be emphasised that this has nothing to do with (heaven forbid) radical idealism. And the exclusion of evaluative terms from argument is not being suggested. I am simply pointing towards an aspect of appraisal that is discounted in the methodological texts most nurse reviewers are exposed to.

> To describe the concentration camps *sine ira* [without anger] is not to be "objective", but to condone them ... a description of the camps as Hell on earth is more "objective", that is, more adequate to their essence ...
>
> *(Arendt, 2003 [1953], p. 159 – italicisation in original)*

While the natural and mathematical sciences determine facts about the world in comparatively non-evaluative ways, nurse reviewers are predominantly concerned with questions pertaining to people and human interaction. Research with or on humans (like thinking more generally) is inescapably normative, and values suffuse almost everything written about people as opposed to bodies. This much is known. However, the significance of the interpretative problems generated by expressions of value remain underexplored.

Disappointingly, values discussion easily becomes embroiled or conflated with simplistic objective-subjective distinctions. This is regrettable for, as Arendt (2003) makes clear (above), objectivity need not preclude the use of evaluative terms and, indeed, objectivity may in some instances require their use. Objective in this sense references an important element in communication. Specifically, it is appropriate and objective to describe concentration camps using descriptors such as 'Hell' because evocative language of this sort accurately identifies something vital about those camps, something that would be lost if this term was not applied. Likewise, 'callous' might fittingly be applied to a nurse who knowingly and without good reason failed to address a patient's distress when it was in her power, capacity and gift to do so. In both instances evaluative descriptors add to and clarify rather than obfuscate or bias what is conveyed, and their use is not subjective where subjective implies understanding that cannot be shared (i.e. is unique and personal, as opposed to commonly available/accessible).

That said, since evaluative terms are important carriers of meaning, reviewers will want to establish that appropriate rather than inappropriate referents are used. However, anyone accessing texts promoting the standard model will be hard pressed to establish how this might occur. The subject is, as noted, all but ignored.

Methodologists clearly have a great deal of work to do here. For, while associating Hell with concentration camps seems reasonable – phrases such as 'social justice' and 'patient choice' can, depending on use, introduce normative associations that are more contestable. Notoriously, one man's plucky freedom fighter is another's deranged terrorist and, likewise (but less theatrically), researchers and scholars who claim healthcare is, for example, 'underfunded', stake out a political position that reviewers may want to test. That is, when an evaluatively charged word such as 'underfunded' is used in argument, reviewers might and perhaps should note that, even if they personally agree with what is expressed, the position advanced, and the facts they give form to, may be interpreted in more than one way. Indeed, disagreement as to the veracity and appropriateness of value laden terms is likely to occur, and when these descriptors contribute to the structure of what is argued, and when the appropriateness of evaluative expression is challenged, the argument in which that value is situated may be damaged.

Mindful of the previously described fact-value distinction, evidence grounded evaluation can in principle proceed without distress when, tautologically, empiric referents exist. For example, while the exact parameters of a disease or illness event can be impossible to pin down in an absolute sense, we might nonetheless say that 'this' set of measurable symptoms and signs signifies (operationalises) that anyone evidencing them has that disease. And, when conducting a literature review, we could conclude that because so many studies of a particular type record confirmatory data/findings that have confidence intervals within agreed limits then – okay – within identified degrees of certainty/uncertainty we can reasonably propose that this rather than that is likely to be the case. However, value referents are different. Empiric considerations hardly apply when these terms are discussed, and although value descriptors thread through the very fabric of communication, outside clear-cut examples (i.e. bar instances when most reasonable people would assuredly say 'yes' or 'no' to the proposed association), the assessment required to establish appropriateness is necessarily subtle.

Problematically, the type of evaluation needed cannot be summarised or collapsed into bullet points for teaching purposes, or organised as mechanistic or instrumental processes. In reviewing a quantitative paper, we can follow what occurred and if all is done well (if, for example, we examine and agree with the tests run), then to that extent, reviewers can accept the findings (Chapter 6). Yet, crucially, replacing 'Hell' with 'abyss' (a thesaural synonym) in Arendt's (2003) quotation radically alters what is conveyed and, similarly, substituting 'insensitive' or 'uncaring' for 'callous' would change (in my view it lessens) the inaction described above. Note, the point made here – emphasising the importance of individual word choices – echoes similar claims made in Chapters 2 and 3 regards to the way ostensibly trivial differences in the phrasing of review objectives and questions can produce big differences in outcomes. The only difference here is that supposedly minor or inconsequential changes in the choice of value descriptors dramatically alters the meaning of what is said and/ or the structure of argument – and the problem for reviewers remains the same, how are they to appraise whether better or worse descriptor choices have been made? Checking and confirming the statistical tests used in quantitative studies is an exercise that trained and competent statisticians can undertake, and (usually) consensus is possible. However, assessing how evaluatively charged words are used is, largely, a peculiarly personal matter. And, absent agreed measures, reviewers are thrown back onto 'gut instinct' or artistry when assessing the appropriateness or defensibility of evaluative referents. Again, this need not be a major issue. Humanity and arts texts can be recruited to clarify, describe and possibly explain (if not resolve) the issues involved. Nonetheless, given the pivotal role that values play in scientific and scholarly writing, the difficulty that evaluation raises demands more attention than it has hitherto received.

Moving on, if we accept Arendt's (2003) claim (above), reviewers nonetheless need to be careful about what this conception of objective does and does not entail. Mundanely, accepting Arendt's (2003) proposition clearly does not sanction the indiscriminate use of evaluative terms in papers or reviews. These terms and the judgements they exhibit are, to repeat, integral to communication. However, more interestingly, we must be wary of jumping to the unwarranted inference that, insofar as value referents communicate or tell us about how things are, value exists in the world. That is, granting that evaluative terms and values they describe carry objective weight (in Arendt's sense) raises the lid on theories of normative motivation.

This subject has an extensive and developed literature, it can be approached in many ways, and the following brief comments cannot hope to do justice to the topic. Nevertheless, in crude synopsis, normative motivation describes opposed arguments about why we act (are caused to act). Thus, focusing simply on moral reasoning, do humans form desires and beliefs about what is good and bad (right and wrong) that thereafter prompt them to interpret the world and act (behave) in certain ways? Or, are motivating (action initiating) desires-beliefs generated in reaction to (in acknowledgement of) objective states of affair regarding what exists and is good or bad in the world? In the first instance humans determine moral meaning, in the second, moral meaning is recognised as emanating or existing outside human determination. Rephrased, internalists hold that moral value, and the desires and beliefs accompanying value, are subjective human constructions. That is, value is made or given by us, and nothing is good or bad independently of human resolve (i.e. nothing is good or bad in or of itself). Externalists, however, reject this view. They hold that moral values reference good and bad in the world. That is, events can be good or bad even if 'we' (humanity) do not individually and/or collectively acknowledge them as such.

Earlier chapters suggested that reviewers should think about the ways in which their own beliefs-values influence location and appraisal. It was suggested that if these beliefs-values were understood they might, potentially, contribute positively to the review process. Here it is proposed that reviewers need to sensitise themselves to the existence and role played by values in argument, and when appropriate, they need to question and debunk unsustainable claims. This, however, demands that a critical stance be maintained in relation to those values (Arendt's spectator metaphor in contemplation is appropriate here). Arts and humanity literatures may support and enable this endeavour, and to be successful, it is likely that a contemplative rather than instrumental approach to reviews will be required in some if not all instances. Further, while the following statements rest principally on personal experience, overly declarative claims – which may be associated with externalist 'like' expression – hampers this process. Thus, when the 'obvious' correctness of particular forms of, for example, healthcare financing and organisation is assumed, and when the 'obvious' moral wickedness and intellectual duplicity of those favouring alternative approaches to those 'we' favour is supposed, the status or location of such obviousness needs to be clarified. That is, reviewers should ask: are the values expressed correct because that is how it seems to whoever advocates for them, or are those judgements correct in some other (external) sense? If a value position is correct in someone's opinion then it is open to challenge and possible rebuttal. However, if a value is claimed as 'correct', if its moral rightness is placed outside of or beyond question, then either debate and challenge must end, or those who accept and reject whatever position is in play will stop communicating.

Rather than seeing values as a problem to be 'got around', if the contribution made by values to argumentative structure and reasoning is realised – and this probably necessitates incorporating ideas derived from humanity and arts scholarship into the reviews nurses conduct – then the contribution of values to communication can be highlighted. Potentially, benefit (improved or at least more stimulating reviews) might derive from recognising and emphasising the part played by values in understanding. But, if it is supposed that values are necessarily troublesome, if we presume their influence must be minimised or expunged, then this positive role cannot be known. Like other facets of the review process – and this is clearly a leitmotif of the book – more work needs to be undertaken if reviewers are to be enabled to engage with these issues in a sensible and productive manner.

An unthinking focus on action

Arguments presented above concerning values, the potential inclusion of humanity and arts texts in reviews, contemplation as a good in and of itself and, indeed, all other matters – rest on or incorporate two assumptions. First, parochialism is generally unhelpful (we almost always need to look beyond disciplinary boundaries). And, second, nurse reviewers can and should read widely. Both these premises in turn sit on the idea that reviews – indeed nursing – require, to be maximally beneficial, those who undertake this activity and role to engage critically at a reasonably 'deep' level with what it is that they do.

Chapter 1, however, suggested that reading in the context of reviews is often undervalued by nursing students, educators and researchers. The assertion was not quantified (only anecdotal evidence was provided in support of the claim) and it clearly applies, if it applies at all, to some rather than all nurses. Nonetheless, where it exists, the disposition to undervalue reading presumably impacts negatively on how reviews are approached and conducted (it, for example, feeds parochialism). Suggestions as to why this disposition exists are perforce provisional. However, first, recruits might be attracted to the profession because, among other positives, it is or likes to portray itself as being action orientated. Indeed, stressing the 'practice based' nature of nursing might – though it need not – preference action over the cognitive or intellectual components of activity (see previous arguments regards recruitment) and, perhaps, this focus presents a skewed image of nursing.

Thus, nurses act in the world to enable positive ends. This acting requires psycho-motor skills, technical expertise and, almost always, sophisticated forms of critical/cognitive functioning. Reading and contemplation contribute to understanding and, hence, effective nursing. However, insofar as reading and contemplation involve or necessitate stepping back from the hurly-burly of ongoing clinical bustle (Arendt's 'withdrawal') it is unsurprising that, when providing hands-on care, these activities fall into abeyance. Bulleted guidelines and notes are all that can be consumed amidst the swirl or melee of everyday practice – and as Chapter 1 records, absent 'set aside' or dedicated within work reading time, clinicians cannot engage with anything other than these reduced sources. This is true of practice. Yet nursing's 'action focus' may also impact detrimentally (if unwittingly) on under- and postgraduate students undertaking college or academic work.

By this I mean, while it might be supposed that reading and reviews could be progressed in a more thorough and considered fashion outside the clinical environment, this is not necessarily achieved, wanted or encouraged. For example, the need to inculcate correct procedures (e.g. knowing how and where to place ECG leads) often pushes pre- and post-registration (licence) skills education to adopt behaviourally orientated teaching strategies. These approaches can be effective and efficient. However, potentially at least, educators who rely on behaviourist pedagogies may, confronted by time pressures and bloated curriculums, direct students to only read and memorise simple protocols (tick lists) detailing 'right' action.

Clearly this approach to teaching/learning need not downplay critical engagement. However, it can do so and, arguably, similar issues may be experienced in modules and/or courses with more theoretical agendas. Thus, it could be that nursing's action orientation also invests the relationship some nurses have with research and scholarship, and if this is the case, similarly reduced reading expectations might be established. For example, since at any one time a 'right way' of performing skills is generally believed to exist (and these beliefs are frequently and soundly evidence based), it is reasonable to direct students to adopt approved rather than unapproved practices. Further, vis-à-vis skills teaching, discussion and debate regards alternative approaches (i.e. those with an inferior or no evidence base) may be closed down or discouraged. This is understandable. However, if the presence of 'correct procedure' can make skills education decidedly dogmatic, when theoretical modules/courses are pursued, elements of dogmatism might unexpectedly linger.

Thus, those who perform reviews in accordance with the standard model may presume that if 'correct' procedures are followed, defendable or 'right' (evidence based) answers will be found. For this presumption to hold particular types of question must be asked (answerable questions) and particular forms of evidence should be sought (i.e. research reports and systematic reviews of research reports). As argued, this approach to review construction drastically restricts what is read and considered (e.g. non-experimental studies and non-research texts generally find themselves excluded from evaluation). Further, if or when this collapse in reading material and ambition is sanctioned and encouraged by educators, reviews following the model resemble, I suggest, what occurs in some skills teaching.

The standard model's formulaic approach to location and appraisal is attractive to students, educators and novice researchers because it gives the appearance of offering clarity about what is required and, hence, a modicum of (misplaced) confidence in what is concluded. Confidence is important. Nursing claims the title of profession because, in part, the actions of its members are supposedly evidence based, and reviews grounded on the standard model contribute to this base without necessitating that students or researchers read outside a tightly constrained spectrum of material. Nurse reviewers, moreover, happily comply with standard model conventions because nursing's action orientation is interpreted as necessitating this thing. Put another way, to justify action (to secure an evidence base) nurse reviewers may assume the same inflexible or highly structured stance to engaging with literature to that encapsulated in behaviourally orientated skills teaching and this, feasibly, encourages or facilitates a disengagement from wide reading.

Second, at the time of writing, my institution accepts recruits who achieve three Cs at A level or equivalent. Arguably, these are not high entry requirements, and with 'relevant' work experience lesser grades are considered at clearing. Further, if or insofar as past grade attainment predicts future academic potential, and to the extent that academic potential correlates with or reflects an aptitude for reading/critical thinking, it may be that we are taking in students who are likely to find reading extended or complex texts challenging. This is a troubling topic to discuss. There is clearly nothing set or determined about student ability, and many people who attain poor or disappointing results in secondary (high) school can and do excel at university. On the other hand, students who come from backgrounds that do not embrace reading, and students who have and continue to find academic work difficult are unlikely to engage with anything other than 'reduced' search and review processes. In such circumstances, educators may find themselves pushed to redesign assignments in ways that facilitate or help students complete modules they would otherwise fail. This is not in itself bad. Indeed, revisiting what and how we teach is often beneficial and sensible. However, the worry remains that, perhaps, the redesigns undertaken lead to a diminution in standards and, again, this may involve reducing reading expectations.

In higher education, reading – if taken seriously – references a critical and contemplative encounter with the thoughts of others. This encounter may involve a revaluation, an upturning, of beliefs and values. Reading can therefore be challenging. It is potentially disruptive. It requires focus and practice. And developing and honing the 'skills' involved take effort and time. Arguably, while all students can improve their abilities consequent to education, when nurses have so many things to do and learn, few students will attain the level of proficiency necessary for achieving meaningful competence in the performance of literature reviews, and it is possibly unfair and unreasonable to expect that all do so. Of course, this somewhat negative assessment need not apply to the self-selecting group of nurses who go on to postgraduate and higher studies, and it clearly should not apply to educators and researchers. Nonetheless, as per Chapter 1, expectations and norms regarding reading and review practices established in the early or formative years of education might not be dropped simply with time's passage.

Concluding comments

> Why are we reading, if not in hope of beauty laid bare, life heightened and its deepest mystery probed?
>
> *(Dillard, 1989)*

A great deal more could be said, and I am acutely aware of inconsistencies and blind spots in the arguments presented in this book. However, we end with these last observations. While writing these concluding paragraphs I have, over the last few days, spoken with students, educators and early career researchers. One undergraduate student I spent time with excels in academic work and (I choose to think) she might be open to at least some of the ideas out-lined here. Another, however, struggles with coursework – and while I anticipate that she will eventually complete (be registered/licenced), if current trends persist, every assignment will require multiple rewrites and resubmissions before this occurs. For this student, and many others, much of what is said here must appear idealistic. Indeed, a great deal will seem absurd. Further, as a colleague (educator) stated, 'we simply don't have time for this'. And, to meet the requirements and expectations of funding bodies and editors, career researchers, when performing reviews, 'just do what's necessary'. In these instances, questions such as 'why are we reading' cannot but take an instrumental turn, and 'beauty laid bare' is unlikely to form a major driver for activity.

This is how it is. However, if reviews are worth doing, if we truly want to learn from the literature (or literatures), if this activity can enhance patient care and bolster research findings, while the arguments described here will not appeal to everyone, location and appraisal deserve our consideration. A great deal of what is done by students, educators and researchers has, to repeat earlier comments, merit. Nonetheless, improvement is possible, and at a minimum, supportive and standalone reviews undertaken by nurses (including many that are published) could frequently be refined. Faced with the 'problem' of reviews, this book asks rather than answers questions and, admittedly, this is frustrating. Moreover, complex issues are grazed rather than plumbed. Yet, hopefully, despite the superficiality that accompanies so general a text, I trust that something worthwhile has been said. And, as ever, I look forward to continued debate into and around this most fascinating of subjects.

Notes

1 Refugee, philosopher, political theorist, historian, journalist, social commentator and activist – Arendt lived through, participated in, and tried to comprehend the twentieth century's 'big events'. A prolific writer, Arendt explored power, authority and evil across works that include but are not limited to; *The Origins of Totalitarianism* (1994 [1951]), *The Human Condition* (1998 [1958]), *Between Past and Future* (2006 [1961]), *Eichmann in Jerusalem: A Report on the Banality of Evil* (2006 [1963]), *On Revolution* (2016 [1963]), and the posthumously edited *The Life of the Mind* (1981 [1978]). Many of these books have convoluted publication histories, and the Hannah Arendt Centre (hac.bard.edu/) is an excellent source of information regards untangling these histories.
2 Page numbers refer to book one of *The Life of the Mind* (1971).
3 While he speaks to different issues and uses alternative language, Ricoeur (2007), in stating that "The conscience that judges denounces the violence of the man of conviction" (p. 55), articulates some-thing of what Arendt means here.
4 While Rolfe's (2010) argument concerning the significance and importance of correctly reading and citing primary sources runs out beyond the immediate point being made, it is worth noting that references in nurse writing too often misconstrue and mangle what authors originally said and/or intended. This topic, this problem, demands further attention.

5 Bennett (2001) recognises the "ethical and political potential within suffering" (p. 160), and Ricoeur (2007) notes that "Some come to see an educative and purgative value in suffering" (p. 71). These statements reference ideas allied to rather than synonymous with those lodged in Huxley (2007). Nonetheless, the point here, supportive humanities materials are (whatever one thinks of these proposals) readily sourced.

6 The work is not or not 'merely' a phenomenology of sort lodged in nursing journals.

7 Despite its venerable age, at the time of writing I can find no reference in the nursing literature to the *Einstellung* effect (Luchins, 1942). This refers to the propensity of humans to fixate or settle on one solution to a problem and – once an explanation or idea becomes established – alternative 'better' solutions are ignored/pass unrecognised (Thomas, Didierjean and Kuhn, 2018). This psychological phenomenon, which influences experts and novices alike, might potentially be recruited to explain numerous aspects of the way in which the standard model of reviews (as described in this book) has been adopted. More specifically, the mechanism 'behind' bias associated with cherry picking feasibly rests, in part, on something like this effect.

REFERENCES

A Guide to Active Citation – Version 1.1 for Pilot Projects (January 2013). Available online: www.prince ton.edu/~amoravcs/library/guide_active_citation.pdf (accessed 13.02.19).

Achilleas T and Felmont, III F E (2016) What is Wrong With Systematic Reviews and Meta-Analysis: If You Want the Right Answer, Ask the Right Question. *Aesthetic Surgery*. 36(10), 1198–1201.

Achinstein P (2001) *The Book of Evidence*. Oxford: Oxford University Press.

Achinstein P (2010) *Evidence, Explanation, and Realism: Essays in Philosophy of Science*. Oxford: Oxford University Press.

Adams L (2017) Women in Scotland allowed abortion pill at home. *BBC News – Scotland*. Report dated 26.10.17. Available online: www.bbc.co.uk/news/uk-scotland-41760959 (accessed 27.02.19).

Aiken L H, Cerón C, Simonetti M, Lake E T, Galiano A, Garbarini A, Soto P, Bravo D, and Smith H L (2018) Hospital Nurse Staffing And Patient Outcomes. *Revista Médica Clínica Las Condes*. 29(3), 322–327.

Aiken L H, Sloane D M, Luk Bruyneel M S, Van den Heede K, Griffiths P, Busse R, Diomidous M, Kinnunen J, Kózka M, Lesaffre E, McHugh M D, Moreno-Casbas M T, Rafferty A M, Schwendi-mann R, Scott A P, Tishelman C, van Achterberg T, and Sermeus W (2014) Nurse staffing and education and hospital mortality in nine European countries: a retrospective observational study. *The Lancet*. 383(9931), 1824–1830.

Aimee M (2017) Subjective from the start: a critique of transformative criticism. *Nursing Philosophy*. 18(2), 1–5.

Alame D (2018) How Should Clinicians Weigh the Benefits and Harms of Discussing Politicized Topics that Influence Their Individual Patients' Health? *AMA Journal of Ethics*. 19(12), 1174–1182.

Alligood M R and Fawcett J (2017) The Theory of the Art of Nursing and the Practice of Human Care Quality. *Visions*. 23(1), 4–12.

Allsop J (1995) *Health Policy and the NHS Towards 2000*, 2nd edition. Harlow: Longman Group Limited.

Alper B S and Haynes R B (2016) EBHC pyramid 5.0 for assessing preappraised evidence and guidance. *Evidence-Based Medicine*. 21(4). Available online: http://ebm.bmj.com/content/21/4/123.short (accessed 11.02.19).

Althuis M D and Weed D L (2013) Evidence mapping: methodologic foundations and application to intervention and observational research on sugar-sweetened beverages and health outcomes. *American Journal of Clinical Nutrition*. 98(3), 755–768.

Altman D G (1994). The scandal of poor medical research. *British Medical Journal*. 308, 283–284.

Alving B E, Christensen J B, and Thrysøe L (2018) Hospital nurses' information retrieval behaviours in relation to evidence based nursing: a literature review. *Health Information and Libraries Journal*. 35(1), 3–23.

Ameling A (2000) Prayer: An Ancient Healing Practice Becomes New Again. *Holistic Nursing Practice*. 14(3), 40–49.

Anderson E (2004) Uses of Value Judgements in Science: A General Argument, with Lessons from a Case Study of Feminist Research on Divorce. *Hypatia*. 19(1), 1–24.

Andrew-Perez J, Poon C C Y, Merrifield R D, Wong S T C, and Yang G-Z (2015) Big Data for Health. *IEEE Journal of Biomedical and Health Informatics*. 19(4), 1193–1208.

Archer M S (1995) *Realist Social Theory: The Morphogenetic Approach*. Cambridge: Cambridge University Press.

Arendt H (2016) *On Revolution*, paperback edition. London: Faber and Faber.

Arendt H (2006) *Between Past and Future: Eight Exercises in Political Thought*. London: Penguin Books.

Arendt H (2006) *Eichmann in Jerusalem: A Report on the Banality of Evil*. London: Penguin Books.

Arendt H (2003) A Reply to Eric Voegelin. In *The Portable Hannah Arendt*. London: Penguin Books.

Arendt H (1998) *The Human Condition*, 2nd edition. London: University of Chicago Press.

Arendt H (1994) *The Origins of Totalitarianism*. London: Penguin Books.

Arendt H (1978) *The Life of the Mind*, one-volume edition. New York: Harvest Books.

Aristotle (2009) *The Nicomachean Ethics*. Oxford: Oxford University Press.

Arnold M (2009) [1869] *Culture and Anarchy*. Oxford: Oxford University Press.

Artino A R, Phillips A W, Utrankar A, Ta A Q, and Durning S J (2018) "The Questions Shape the Answers": Assessing the Quality of Published Survey Instruments in Health Professions Education Research. *Academic Medicine*. 93(3), 456–463.

Athey S and Imbens G (2015) Recursive Partitioning for Heterogeneous Causal Effects. Working paper. Available online: www.researchgate.net/profile/Guido_Imbens/publication/274644919_Machine_Lea rning_Methods_for_Estimating_Heterogeneous_Causal_Effects/links/553c02250cf2c415bb0b1720.pdf (accessed 09.12.18).

Atkins S, Lewis S, Smith H, Engel M, Fretheim A, and Volmink J (2008) Conducting a meta-ethnography of qualitative literature: lessons learnt. *BMC Medical Research Methodology*. 8(21). Available online: https://bm cmedresmethodol.biomedcentral.com/track/pdf/10.1186/1471-2288-8-21?site=bmcmedresmeth odol.biomedcentral.com (accessed 21.10.18).

Aubeeluck A, Stacey G, and Stupple E J N (2016) Do graduate entry nursing student's experience 'Imposter Phenomenon'?: An issue for debate. *Nurse Education in Practice*. 19(4), 104–106.

Austgard K I (2008) What characterises nursing care? A hermeneutical philosophical inquiry. *Scandinavian Journal of Caring Science*. 22(2), 314–319.

Aveyard H (2018) *Doing a Literature Review in Health and Social Care: A Practical Guide*. Fourth Edition. Maidenhead: McGraw Hill – Open University Press.

Aveyard H and Sharp P (2013) *A Beginner's Guide to Evidence-Based Practice in Health and Social Care*. Second edition. Maidenhead: McGraw-Hill Education – Open University Press.

Aveyard H, Payne S, and Preston N (2016) *A Post-graduate's Guide to Doing a Literature Review in Health and Social Care*. Maidenhead: McGraw Hill – Open University Press.

Ayala R A (2018) Invited Commentary: Thinking of conceptual reviews and systematic reviews. *Nursing Inquiry*. 25(4), 1–2.

Bacon F (1999) *The Essays or Counsels: Civil and Moral*. Oxford: Oxford University Press.

Baillie L (2017) An exploration of the 6Cs as a set of values for nursing practice. *British Journal of Nursing*. 26(10), 558–563.

Baldi H, Lago E D, De Bardi S, Sartor G, Soriani N, Zanotti R, and Gregori D (2014) Trends in RCT nursing research over 20 years: mind the gap. *British Journal of Nursing*. 23(16), 895–899.

Banner D, Janke F, and King-Shier K (2016) Making evidence-based practice happen in 'real world' contexts: the importance of collaborative partnerships. In Lipscomb M (ed.) *Exploring Evidence-Based Practice: Debates and Challenges in Nursing*, pp. 11–28. London: Routledge.

Barroso J, Gollop C J, Sandelowski M, Meynell J, Pearce P, and Collins L J (2003) The challenge of searching for and retrieving qualitative studies. *Western Journal of Nursing Research*. 25(2), 153–178.

Barker J (2013) *Evidence-based Practice for Nurses*, 2nd edition. London: Sage.

Barkway P (2001) Michael Crotty and nursing phenomenology: Criticism or critique? *Nursing Inquiry.* 8(3), 191–195.

Bareinboim E (2014) Generalizability in Causal Inference: Theory and Algorithms. UCLA Electronic Theses and Dissertations. Available online: https://escholarship.org/content/qt1427f0kt/qt1427f0kt.pdf (accessed 12.02.19).

Barnett R and Coate K (2005) *Engaging the Curriculum in Higher Education.* Series: The Society for Research into Higher Education. Berkshire: Open University Press – McGraw-Hill Education.

Barrow J D (1998) *Impossibility: The Limits of Science and the Science of Limits.* Oxford: Oxford University Press.

Bates M J (1989) The design of browsing and berry picking techniques for the online search interface. *Online Review.* 13(5), 407–423.

Bazian (2016) Heart attacks linked to media statins reports … reports media. Behind the Headlines – blog: 29.06.2016. Available online: www.nhs.uk/news/heart-and-lungs/heart-attacks-linked-to-media-statin-reports-reports-media/ (accessed 12.01.19).

Belluz J (2016) This is why you shouldn't believe that exciting new medical study. *Vox.* Published 19.10.16. Available online: www.vox.com/2015/3/23/8264355/research-study-hype (accessed 31.10.18).

Bench S, Day T, and Metcalfe A (2013) Randomised controlled trials: an introduction for nurse researchers. *Nurse Researcher.* 20(5), 38–44.

Bennett J (2001) *The Enchantment of Modern Life: Attachments, Crossings, and Ethics.* Princeton: Princeton University Press.

Berger R (2015) Now you see it, now I don't: researcher's position and reflexivity in qualitative research. *Qualitative Research.* 15(2), 219–234.

Berlin I (1998a) [1953] Historical Inevitability. In Hardy H and Hausheer R (eds) *The Proper Study of Mankind: An Anthology of Essays*, pp. 119–190. London: Pimlico – Random House.

Berlin I (1998b) [1960] The concept of scientific history. In Hardy H and Hausheer R (eds) *The Proper Study of Mankind: An Anthology of Essays*, pp. 17–58. London: Pimlico – Random House.

Berlin I (1998c) [1973] The counter-enlightenment. In Hardy H and Hausheer R (eds) *The Proper Study of Mankind: An Anthology of Essays*, pp. 243–268. London: Pimlico – Random House.

Bernier R, Halpin E, Staffa S J, Benson L, DiNardo J A, and Nasr V G (2018) Inclusion of non-English-speaking patients in research: A single institution experience. *Pediatric Anesthesia.* 28(5), 415–420.

Bernstein R J (2010) *The Pragmatic Turn.* Cambridge: Polity Press.

Bhaskar R (1997) *A Realist Theory of Science.* London: Verso Classics.

Bickford C J (2017) The Professional Association's Perspective on Nursing Informatics and Competencies in the US. In Murphy J, Goossen W, and Weber P (eds) *Forecasting Informatics Competencies for Nurses in the Future of Connected Health – Studies in Health Technology and Informatics*, pp. 62–68. Available online: http://ebooks.iospress.nl/volume/forecasting-informatics-competencies-for-nurses-in-the-future-of-connected-health-proceedings-of-the-nursing-informatics-post-conference-2016 (accessed 05.10.18).

Bloch M (1976) [1954] *The Historian's Craft.* Manchester: Manchester University Press.

Bluhm R (2017) Nursing theory, social theory, and philosophy of science. In Lipscomb M (ed.) *Social Theory and Nursing*, pp. 35–47. London: Routledge.

Bluhm R (2016) Evidence-based nursing and the generalizability of research results. In Lipscomb M (ed.) *Exploring Evidence-Based Practice: Debates and Challenges in Nursing*, pp. 88–98. London: Routledge.

Bluhm R (2014) The (dis)unity of nursing science. *Nursing Philosophy.* 15(4), 250–260.

Boell S K and Cezec-Kecmanovic D (2014) A Hermeneutic Approach for Conducting Literature Reviews and Literature Searches. *Communications of the Association for Information Systems.* 12–34(1), 257–286.

Boell S K and Cezec-Kecmanovic D (2011) Conference paper: Are systematic reviews better, less biased and of higher quality? *European Conference on Information Systems 2011.* Paper 223. Available online: http://aisel.aisnet.org/ecis2011/223/ (accessed 21.12.18).

Bond E J (1983) *Reason and Value.* Cambridge: Cambridge University Press.

Booth A (2008) Unpacking your literature search toolbox: on search styles and tactics. *Health Information and Libraries Journal.* 25(4), 313–317.

Booth A, Papaioannou D, and Sutton A (2012) *Systematic Approaches to a Successful Literature Review.* London: Sage.

Boutron I and Ravaud P (2018) Misrepresentation and distortion of research in biomedical literature. *Proceedings of the National Academy of Sciences of the United States of America – PNAS.* 115(11), 2613–2619.

Bowling A (2009) *Research Methods in Health: Investigating Health and Health Services,* 3rd edition. Maidenhead: McGraw Hill-Open University Press.

Brannan M J, Fleetwood S, O'Mahoney J, and Vincent S (2017) Critical Essay: Meta-Analysis: A critical realist critique and alternative. *Human Relations.* 70(1), 11–39.

Brekelmans G, Maassen S, Poell R F, Weststrate J, and Geurdes E (2016) Factors influencing nurse participation in continuing professional development: Survey results from the Netherlands. *Nurse Education Today.* 40, 13–19.

Brembs B (2018) Prestigious Science Journals Struggle to Reach Even Average Reliability. *Frontiers in Human Neuroscience.* 12(37). Available online: www.frontiersin.org/articles/10.3389/fnhum.2018. 00037/full?utm_content=bufferfe7ed&utm_medium=social&utm_source=facebook.com&utm_ campaign=buffer (accessed 12.11.18).

Brett S (2018) Generalizability in qualitative research: misunderstandings, opportunities and recommendations for the sport and exercise sciences. *Qualitative Research in Sport, Exercise and Health.* 10(1), 137–149.

Briggs W M (2017) The substitute for p-Values. *Journal of the American Statistical Association.* 112(519), 897–898.

Britten N, Garside R, Pope C, Frost J, and Cooper C (2017) Asking More of Qualitative Synthesis: A Response to Sally Thorne…Thorne S. Metasynthetic Madness: What Kind of Monster Have We Created? *Qualitative Health Research.* 27(9), 1370–1376.

Broom M, Mahoney E, and Sellman D (2017) Evidence-Based Practice. In Sellman D and Snelling P (eds) *Becoming A Nurse: Fundamentals Of Professional Practice For Nursing,* 2nd edition. London: Routledge.

Brown A W, Kaiser K A, and Allison D B (2018) Issues with data and analysis: Errors, underlying themes, and potential solutions. *Proceedings of the National Academy of Sciences of the United States of America – PNAS.* 115(11), 2563–2570.

Brown C G (2015) Success Is Not final! Onward to the Future of Evidence-Based Practice. *Clinical Journal of Oncology Nursing.* 19(2), 146–147.

Brown S L, Whiting D, Fielden H G, Saini P, Beesley H, Holcombe C, Holcombe S, Greenhalgh L, Fairburn L, and Salmon P (2017) Qualitative analysis of how patients decide that they want risk-reducing mastectomy, and the implications for surgeons in responding to emotionally-motivated patient requests. *PLoS ONE* 12(5): e0178392. Available online: http://journals.plos.org/plosone/a rticle?id=10.1371/journal.pone.0178392 (accessed 20.11.18).

Butun A and Hemingway P (2018) A qualitative systematic review of the reasons for parental attendance at the emergency department with children presenting with minor illness. *International Emergency Nursing.* 36, 56–62.

Cai L, Tian J, Liu J, Bai X, Lee I, Kong X, and Xia F (2019) Scholarly impact assessment: a survey of citation weighting solutions. *Scientometrics.* 118(2), 453–478.

Camus A (2013) [1951] *The Rebel.* London: Penguin Books.

Canagarajah S (2005) Rhetoricizing reflexivity. *Journal of Language, Identity and Education.* 4(4), 309–315.

Carnap R (2003) [1928] Der logische Aufbau der Welt (1928 – Berlin: Weltkreis) English translation – *The Logical Structure of the World.* Translation. R. George. Chicago: Open Court Classics.

Carruthers P (2013) *The Opacity of Mind: An Integrative Theory of Self-Knowledge.* Oxford: Oxford University Press.

Castañeda O J M (2019) (Un)contested evidence: scientific literature, systematic reviews and the politics of evidence in the introduction of HPV vaccines in Colombia. *Sociology of Health and Illness.* 41(1), 81–94.

Chatfield T (2017) Podcast: Tom Chatfield on Critical Thinking and Bias. *Social Science Bites.* Available online: http://socialsciencebites.libsyn.com/tom-chatfield-on-critical-thinking-and-bias (accessed 12.10.18).

Chignell A (2018) The Ethics of Belief. *The Stanford Encyclopedia of Philosophy.* Spring 2018 edition. Editor Zalta E N. Available online: https://plato.stanford.edu/entries/ethics-belief/ (accessed 23.12.18).

Choi S W and Cheung (2016) Don't judge a book by its cover, don't judge a study by its abstract. Common statistical errors seen in medical papers. *Anaesthesia.* 71(7), 843–845.

Chomsky N (2014) Science, Mind, and the Limits of Understanding. The Science and Faith Foundation (STOQ), The Vatican, January 2014. Available online: https://chomsky.info/201401__/ (accessed 28.07.18).

Christmals C D and Gross J J (2017) An Integrative Literature Review Framework For Postgraduate Nursing Research Reviews. *European Journal of Research in Medical Sciences.* 5(1), 7–15.

Clarke S, Clark-Burg K, and Pavlos E (2018) Clinical handover of immediate post-operative patients: A literature review. *The Journal of Perioperative Nursing in Australia.* 31(2), 29–35.

Clifford W K (2018) [1877] *The Ethics of Belief.* Available online: www.memelyceum.com/documents/ethics_of_belief.pdf (accessed 23.12.18).

Coakley A B, Barron A-M, and Annese C D (2016). Exploring the experience and impact of therapeutic touch treatments for nurse colleagues. *Visions: The Journal of Rogerian Nursing Science.* 22(1), Manuscript 1. Available online: http://web.b.ebscohost.com.proxy.worc.ac.uk/ehost/pdfviewer/pdfviewer?vid=18&sid=284cbbd0-860c-4c5b-abe3-e951cf0435ff%40pdc-v-sessmgr01 (accessed 22.11.18).

Cochrane Library (2018) About Cochrane Reviews. Available online: www.cochranelibrary.com/about/about-cochrane-reviews (accessed 21.12.18).

Cochrane Community (2017) Cochrane Knowledge Translation Framework – April 2017. Available online: https://community.cochrane.org/sites/default/files/uploads/Cochrane%20Knowledge%20Translation%20Framework%281%29.pdf (accessed 27.11.18).

Cohn E G, Jia H, and Larson E (2009) Evaluation of statistical approaches in quantitative nursing research. *Clinical Nursing Research.* 18(3), 223–241.

Collingridge D S and Gantt E E (2008) The Quality of Qualitative Research. *American Journal of Medical Quality.* 23(5), 389–395.

Collini S (2012) *What Are Universities For?* London: Penguin Books.

Cooper A (2017) Blog: A Nurse who has 'Sold her Soul'? Available online: https://anniecoops.com/2017/09/20/a-nurse-who-has-sold-her-soul/ (accessed 21.09.18).

Cope V, Jones B, and Hendricks J (2016) Resilience as resistance to the new managerialism: portraits that reframe nursing through quotes from the field. *Journal of Nursing Management.* 24(1), 115–122.

Cottrell S (2005) *Critical Thinking Skills: Developing Effective Analysis and Argument.* Basingstoke: Palgrave Macmillan.

Coughlan M and Cronin P (2017) *Doing A Literature Review In Nursing, Health And Social Care.* London: Sage.

Cowan R (2015) Cognitive Penetrability and Ethical Perception. *The Review of Philosophy and Psychology.* 6(4), 665–682.

Cowman S (2017) Editorial – Bedside to bench: re-thinking nursing research. *Journal of Advanced Nursing.* 74(2), 235–236.

Creswell J W (1998) *Qualitative Inquiry and Research Design: Choosing Among Five Traditions.* London: Sage.

Cronin P, Ryan F, and Coughlan M (2008) Undertaking a literature review a step-by-step approach. *British Journal of Nursing.* 17(1), 38–43.

Cumming G (2014) The New Statistics: Why and How. *Psychological Science.* 25(1), 7–29.

Dafoe A (2014) Science Deserves Better: The Imperative to Share Complete Replication Files. *Political Science and Politics.* 47(1), 60–66.

Darbyshire P (2018) Editorial: How not to argue against nursing associates. *Journal of Clinical Nursing.* 27(1–2), 7–8.

Darbyshire P, Thompson D R, and Watson R (2019) Editorial: Nursing Schools: Dumbing down or reaching up? *Journal of Nursing Management.* 27(1), 1–3.

D'Arcy G (2016) Reaching for the starts: RN to BSN. *Nursing.* 46(1), 18–20.

Davies K S (2011) Commentary: Formulating the Evidence Based Practice Question: A Review of the Frameworks. *Evidence Based Library and Information Practice.* 6(2), 75–80. Available online: https://core.ac.uk/download/pdf/25831312.pdf (accessed 12.12.18).

Davies W (2017) *The Limits of Neoliberalism: Authority, Sovereignty and the Logic of Competition.* Revised edition. London: Sage.

Day L, Ziehm S R, Jessup M A, Amedro P, Dawson-Rose C, Derouin A, Kennedy B B, Manahan S, Parish A L, and Remen R N (2017) The power of nursing: An innovative course in values clarification and self-discovery. *Journal of Professional Nursing.* 33(4), 267–270.

Day-Calder M (2017) Show you have the right attitude for the job. *Nursing Standard.* 31(34), 35–36.

Daylight T B (2017) 'The difficulty is the point': teaching spoon-fed students how to really read. *The Guardian.* Saturday 23 December – 22.37 GMT. Available online www.theguardian.com/books/2017/dec/24/the-difficulty-is-the-point-teaching-spoon-fed-students-how-to-really-read?CMP=Share_iOSApp_Other&utm_content=buffer5ff98&utm_medium=social&utm_source=twitter.com&utm_campaign=buffer (accessed 04.01.19).

Deakin N (1994) *The Politics of Welfare: Continuities and Change.* Hemel Hempstead: Harvester Wheatsheaf.

DeJong C and Steinbrook R (2018) Continuing Problems With Financial Conflicts of Interest and Clinical Practice Guidelines. *JAMA.* Available online: https://jamanetwork.com/journals/jama internalmedicine/article-abstract/2708190 (accessed 19.12.18).

Demasi M (2018) Statin wars: have we been misled about the evidence? A narrative review. *British Journal of Sports Medicine.* 52(14), 905–909.

Descartes R (2006) [1637] *A Discourse on the Method.* Translation Maclean I. Oxford: Oxford University Press.

Deutscher G (2005) *The Unfolding of Language: The Evolution of Mankind's Greatest Invention.* London: William Heinemann-Random House.

de Vrieze J (2017) Bruno Latour, a veteran of the 'science wars', has a new mission. *Science.* Available online: www.sciencemag.org/news/2017/10/latour-qa (accessed 14.11.18).

de Winter J (2016) *Interests and Epistemic Integrity in Science: A New Framework to Assess Interest Influences in Scientific Research Processes.* Maryland: Lexington Books.

di Bitetti M S and Ferreras J A (2017) Publish (in English) or perish: The effect on citation rate of using languages other than English in scientific publications. *Ambio.* 46(1), 121–127.

Dillard A (1989) Write Till You Drop. Books section. *The New York Times.* May 28, 1989. Available online: https://archive.nytimes.com/www.nytimes.com/books/99/03/28/specials/dillard-drop.html?oref=login (accessed 09.02.19).

Dixon-Woods M, Shaw R L, Agarwal S, and Smith J A (2004) The problem of appraising qualitative research: Developing Research. *Quality and Safety in Healthcare.* 13(3), 223–225.

Djulbegovic B and Guyatt G H (2017) Progress in evidence-based medicine: a quarter century on. *Lancet.* 390(10092), 415–423.

Doyle A C (2018) *The Adventures of Sherlock Holmes.* Vintage Edition. London: Penguin Classics.

Drayton N and Weston K M (2015) Exploring values in nursing: generating new perspectives on clinical practice. *Australian Journal of Advanced Nursing.* 33(1), 14–22.

Dupré J (2001) *Human Nature and the Limits of Science.* Oxford: Oxford University Press.

Dyson S (2018) *Critical Pedagogy in Nursing: Transformational Approaches to Nurse Education in a Globalized World.* London: Palgrave Macmillan.

EASAC (2017) Homeopathic products and practices: assessing the evidence and ensuring consistency in regulating medical claims in the EU. Available online: www.easac.eu/fileadmin/PDF_s/reports_sta tements/EASAC_Homepathy_statement_web_final.pdf (accessed 27.11.17).

Eastwood K J, Boyle M J, Williams B, and Fairhall R (2011) Numeracy skills of nursing students. *Nurse Education Today*. 31(8), 815–818.

EBSCO (2018) EBSCO Nursing Resources – CINAHL Databases. Available online: www.ebscohost. com/nursing/products/cinahl-databases (accessed 10.10.18).

Edwards P K (2017) A realist alternative to meta-analysis. Two papers. *Human Relations*. 70(1), 8–10.

Eisenhart M (2009) Generalization from Qualitative Inquiry. In Ercikan K and Roth W-M (eds) (2009) *Generalization from Educational Research: Beyond Qualitative and Quantitative Polarization*, pp. 51–66. London: Routledge.

Ellis P (2016) Towards an inclusive model of evidence-based care. In Ellis P (ed.) *Evidence-based Practice in Nursing*, 3rd edition. London: Sage.

Elman C, Kapiszewski D, and Vinuela L (2010) Qualitative Data Archiving: Rewards and Challenges. *Political Science and Politics*, 43(1), 23–27.

Epstein B (2015) *The Ant Trap: Rebuilding the Foundations of the Social Sciences*. Oxford: Oxford University Press.

Erdmann T P, De Mast J, and Warrens M J (2015) Some common errors of experimental design, interpretation and inference in agreement studies. *Statistical Methods in Medical Research*. 24(6), 920–935.

Evans M (1998) De-constructing death: In memory of Gillian Rose. *Women: A Cultural Review*. 9(1), 18–33.

Farahnaz S, Azadi T, and Azadi T (2017) Barriers to using electronic evidence based literature in nursing practice: a systematised review. *Health Information and Libraries Journal*. 34(3), 187–199.

Feinstein N W (2015) Education, communication, and science in the public space. *Journal of Research in Science Teaching*. 52(2), 145–163.

Few S (2018) *Big Data, Big Dupe: A Little Book about a Big Bunch of Nonsense*. El Dorado Hills: Bryan Pierce – Analytics Press.

Fileborn B (2017) Sexual Assault and Justice for Older Women: A Critical Review of the Literature. *Trauma, Violence and Abuse*. 18(5), 496–507.

Fendler L (2006) Why Generalizability is not Generalizable. *Journal of Philosophy of Education*. 40(4), 437–449.

Finfgeld-Connett D (2010) Generalizability and transferability of meta-synthesis research findings. *Journal of Advanced Nursing*. 66(2), 246–254.

Finfgeld-Connett D and Johnson E D (2013) Literature search strategies for conducting knowledge-building and theory-generating qualitative systematic reviews. *Journal of Advanced Nursing*. 69(1), 194–204.

Finlay L (2002a) Negotiating the swamp: The opportunity and challenge of reflexivity in research practice. *Qualitative Research*. 2(2), 209–230.

Finlay L (2002b) "Outing" the researcher: The provenance, process, and practice of reflexivity. *Qualitative Health Research*. 12(4), 531–545.

Finlay S (2014) *Predicative Analytics, Data Mining and Big Data: Myths, Misconceptions and Methods*. Basingstoke: Palgrave Macmillan.

Flemming K (2007a) Synthesis of qualitative research and evidence-based nursing. *British Journal of Nursing*. 16(10), 616–620.

Flemming K (2007b) The knowledge base for evidence-based nursing: a role for mixed methods research? *Advances in Nursing Science*. 30(1), 41–51.

Flick U (2008) *Managing Quality in Qualitative Research*. London: Sage.

Foucault M (2002) [1969] *The Archaeology of Knowledge*. Translation by Sheridan Smith A M. London: Routledge.

Frayne S M, Burns R B, Hardt E J, Rosen A K, and Moskowitz M A (1996) The exclusion of non-english-speaking persons from research. *Journal of General Internal Medicine*. 11(1), 39–43.

Freeman T (2006) 'Best practice' in focus group research: making sense of different views. *Journal of Advanced Nursing*. 56(5), 491–497.

Freimuth V S, Jamison A M, An J, Hancock G R, and Quinn S C (2017) Determinants of trust in the flu vaccine for African Americans and Whites. *Social Science and Medicine*. 193, 70–79.

Freshwater D (2004) The appreciation and critique of research findings: skills development. In Freshwater D and Bishop V (eds) (2004) *Nursing Research in Context: Appreciation, Application and Professional Development*, pp. 56–72. Basingstoke: Palgrave Macmillan.

Gaikwad N, Herrera V, and Mickey R W (2019) Text-Based Sources. *American Political Science Association*. Available online: https://papers.ssrn.com/sol3/papers.cfm?abstract_id=3332891 (accessed 26.03.19).

Galdas P (2017) Revisiting bias in qualitative research: Reflections on Its Relationship With Funding and Impact. *International Journal of Qualitative Methods*. 16(1). Available online: http://journals.sagepub.com/doi/full/10.1177/1609406917748992 (accessed 17.12.18).

Gambrill E (2018) [1999] Evidence-based Practice: An Alternative to Authority-based Practice (Revisiting Our Heritage). *Families in Society: The Journal of Contemporary Social Services*. 99(3), 283–294.

Gardiner P (ed.) (1959) *Theories of History. Readings from Classical and Contemporary Sources*. New York: The Free Press – A Division of Macmillan Publishing. Collier Macmillan.

Garrard J (2017) *Health Sciences Literature Review Made Easy: The Matrix Method*. Burlington: Jones and Bartlett Learning.

Garrett B (2018) *Empirical Nursing: The Art of Evidence-Based Care*. Bingley: Emerald Publishing Limited.

Garrett B (2016a) New sophistry: self-deception in the nursing academy. *Nursing Philosophy*. 17(3), 182–193.

Garrett B (2016b) Non-research evidence: What we overlook (but shouldn't). In Lipscomb M (ed.) *Exploring Evidence-Based Practice: Debates and Challenges in Nursing*, pp. 113–131. London: Routledge.

Gaudet J, Singh M D, Epstein I, Santa Mina E, and Gula T (2014) Learn the game but don't play it: Nurses perspectives on learning and applying statistics in practice. *Nurse Education Today*. 34(7), 1080–1086.

Gelman A (2018) How to Think Scientifically about Scientists' Proposals for Fixing Science. *Socius: Sociological Research for a Dynamic World*. 4, 1–2.

George V and Wilding P (1994) *Welfare and Ideology*. Hemel Hempstead: Harvester Wheatsheaf.

Giardina T D, Haskell H, Menon S, Hallisy J, Southwick F S, Sarkar U, Royce K E, and Singh H (2018) Learning From Patients' Experiences Related To Diagnostic Errors Is Essential For Progress In Patient Safety. *Health Affairs*. 37(11), 1821–1827.

Gifford W, Zhang Q, Chen S, Davies B, Xie R, Wen S-W, and Harvey G (2018) When east meets west: a qualitative study of barriers and facilitators to evidence-based practice in Hunan China. *BMC*. 17–26. Available online: https://bmcnurs.biomedcentral.com/articles/10.1186/s12912-018-0295-x (accessed 15.11.18).

Girvin J (2018) Every picture tells a story. Blog post 27.07.18. Available online: https://junegirvin2.wordpress.com/ (accessed 12.12.18).

Glaister K (2007) The presence of mathematics and computer anxiety in nursing students and their effects on medication dosage calculations. *Nurse Education Today*. 27(4), 341–347.

Glaser E (2015) Bureaucracy: why won't scholars break their paper chains? *Times Higher Education*. May 21st. Available online: www.timeshighereducation.com/features/bureaucracy-why-wont-scholars-break-their-paper-chains/2020256.article (accessed 11.09.18).

Glazer S (2001) Therapeutic touch and postmodernism in nursing. *Nursing Philosophy*. 2(3), 196–212.

Glenn D G (2016) Big Data and Pharmacovigilance: The Role of Oncology Nurses. *Clinical Journal of Oncology Nursing*. 20(5), 478–480.

Goh L (2017) Evidence-based health practice: a fairytale or reality. Available online: www.students4bestevidence.net/evidence-based-health-practice-a-fairytale-or-reality/?utm_content=buffer67596&utm_medium=social&utm_source=twitter.com&utm_campaign=buffer (accessed 28.11.18).

Golafshani N (2003) Understanding Reliability and Validity in Qualitative Research. *The Qualitative Report*. 8(4), 597–607.

Goldacre B (2014a) Cherry-Picking Is Bad. At Least Warn Us When You Do It. In *I Think You'll Find It's A Bit More Complicated Than That*, pp. 5–8. London: Fourth Estate.

Goldacre B (2014b) [2011] There's Something Magical About Watching Patterns Emerge from Data. In *I Think You'll Find It's A Bit More Complicated Than That*, pp. 73–75. London: Fourth Estate.

Goldacre B (2012) *Bad Pharma: How Medicine is Broken, and How We Can Fix It*. London: Fourth Estate.

Goldacre B (2011) Foreword. In Evans I, Thornton H, Chalmers I, and Glasziou P *Testing Treatments: Better Research for Better Healthcare*, 2nd edition. London: Pinter & Martin Ltd.

Goldberg S (2012) A Reliabilist Foundationalist Coherentism. *Erkenntnis*. 77(2), 187–196.

Goodell L S, Stage V C, and Cooke N K (2016) Practical Qualitative Research Strategies: Training Interviewers and Coders. *Journal of Nutrition, Education and Behavior*. 48(8), 578–585.

Gorman S E and Gorman J M (2016) *Denying to the Grave: Why We Ignore the Facts that Will Save Us*. Oxford: Oxford University Press.

Gorman T (2001) Gillian Rose and the project of a Critical Marxism. *Radical Philosophy*. 105, 25–36. Available online: www.radicalphilosophy.com/wp-content/files_mf/rp105_article3_gillianroseprojec tofacriticalmarxism_gorman.pdf (accessed 03.01.19).

Graeber D (2015) *The Utopia of Rules: On Technology, Stupidity, and the Secret Joys of Bureaucracy*. London: Melville House Publishing.

Gray J (2009) [1995] *Enlightenment's Wake: Politics and Culture at the Close of the Modern Age*. London: Routledge.

Gray R, Hassanien R N, and Thompson D R (2017) Journal editors and their h-index. *Journal of Advanced Nursing*. 73(9), 2031–2034.

Green A, Jeffs D, Huett A, Jones L R, Schmid B, Scott A R, and Walker L (2014) Increasing Capacity for Evidence-Based Practice Through the Evidence-Based Practice Academy. *Journal of Continuing Education in Nursing*. 45(2), 83–92.

Green S (2018) Science and Journalism In the Age of "Fake News" – Blog post. *The Wiley Network*. Available online: https://hub.wiley.com/community/exchanges/discover/blog/2018/10/25/scien ce-and-journalism-in-the-age-of-fake-news?referrer=exchanges (accessed 20.12.18).

Greenhalgh T (2018) *How to Implement Evidence-Based Healthcare*. Oxford: Wiley Blackwell.

Greenhalgh T (2016) Cultural contexts of health: the use of narrative research in the health sector. Health Evidence Network Synthesis Report 49. Copenhagen: World Health Organisation.

Greenhalgh T (2014) *How to read a paper: The basics of evidence-based medicine*. Oxford: Wiley Blackwell.

Greenhalgh T (2012) Editorial – Why do we always end up here? Evidence-based medicine's conceptual cul-de-sacs and some off-road alternative routes. *Journal of Primary Care*. 4(2), 92–97.

Greenhalgh T (2004). Meta-narrative mapping: A new approach to the systematic review of complex evidence. In Hurwitz B, Greenhalgh T, and Skultans V (eds) *Narrative Research in Health and Illness*, pp. 349–381. Oxford: Blackwell.

Greenhalgh T and Russel J (2009) Evidence-based policy making: a critique. *Perspectives in Biology and Medicine*. 52(2), 304–318.

Greenhalgh T, Thorne S, and Malterud K (2018) Perspective: Time to challenge the spurious hierarchy of systematic over narrative reviews? *European Journal of Clinical Investigation*. 48(6), 1–6.

Griffiths A P (ed.) (1967) *Knowledge and Belief*. Oxford: Oxford University Press.

Guba E G and Lincoln Y S (1998) Competing paradigms in qualitative research. In Denzin N K and Lincoln S Y (eds) *The Landscape of Qualitative Research: Theories and Issues*, pp. 195–220. London: Sage.

Guggenbühl-Craig A (2015) *Power in The Helping Professions*. Translation, M Gubitz. Foreword, J R Haule. Thompson, CN: Spring Publications.

Guttmann A, Schull M J, Vermeulen M J, and Stukel T A (2011) Association between waiting times and short term mortality and hospital admission after departure from emergency department: population based cohort study from Ontario, Canada. *British Medical Journal*. 342. Available online: www. bmj.com/content/342/bmj.d2983.full (accessed 03.10.18).

Guyatt G H (1991) Editorial: Evidence-based medicine. *APC Journal Club Archives*. 114(2), p. A16. Available online: www.acpjc.org/Content/114/2/issue/ACPJC-1991-114-2-A16.htm (accessed 27.11.18).

Haack S (2014) *Evidence Matters: Science, Proof, And Truth In The Law*. Cambridge: Cambridge University Press.

Haddaway N R, Land M, and Macura B (2017) "A little learning is a dangerous thing": A call for better understanding of the term 'systematic review'. *Environmental International.* 99, 356–360.

Hall P A (2016) Transparency, Research Integrity and Multiple Methods. *Comparative Politics Newsletter.* 26(1), 28–31. Available online: https://pdfs.semanticscholar.org/d733/0acec00b6f401d274222cf13d9561a ceb7bb.pdf (accessed 24.11.18).

Hamilton E (2016) Why I became a homeopath. *Health and Homeopathy.* 27.

Hammersley M (2007) The issue of quality in qualitative research. *International Journal of Research and Method in Education.* 30(3), 287–305.

Hannes K (2017) Quality assessment of qualitative research studies in the context of literature reviews: moving smoothly from one decision point to another. In European Congress of Qualitative Inquiry Proceedings 2017, pp. 135–139. February 7–10. Leuven, Belgium. Available online: https://biblio. ugent.be/publication/8511570/file/8513715#page=141 (accessed 01.12.18).

Hannes K and Lockwood C (2011) Pragmatism as the philosophical foundation for the Joanna Briggs meta-aggregative approach to qualitative evidence synthesis. *Journal of Advanced Nursing.* 67(7), 1632–1642.

Hansson S O (2017) Science denial as a form of pseudoscience. *Studies in History and Philosophy of Science Part A.* 63, 39–47.

Hanucharurnkul S and Turale S (2017) Integration: The Uniqueness of Nursing Practice. *Pacific Rim International Journal of Nursing Practice.* 21(2), 93–96.

Harden A and Thomas J (2005) Methodological issues in combining diverse study types in systematic reviews. *International Journal of Social Research Methodology.* 8(3), 257–271.

Hardin R (1982) *Collective Action.* Baltimore: John Hopkins University Press.

Hare R M (1964) *The Language of Morals.* Oxford: Clarendon Press.

Harré R (2009) *Pavlov's Dogs and Schrödinger's Cat: Scenes from the Living Laboratory.* Oxford: Oxford University Press.

Hart L and Little A (2017) Interpreting measures of risk: Translating evidence into practice. *Nurse Practitioner.* 42(2), 50–55.

Harvey C, Thompson S, Pearson M, Willis E, and Toffoli L (2017) Missed nursing care as an 'art form': The contradictions of nurses as carers. *Nursing Inquiry.* 24(3), 8.

Harvey S, Murphy F, Lake R, Jenkins L, Cavanna A, and Tait M (2010) Diagnosing the problem: using a tool to identify pre-registration nursing students' mathematical ability. *Nurse Education in Practice.* 10(3), 119–125.

Hayat M J, Eckardt P, Higgins M, Myoung Jin K, and Schmiege S J (2013) Teaching Statistics to Nursing Students: An Expert Panel Consensus. *Journal of Nursing Education.* 52(6), 330–334.

Heavey E (2015) *Statistics for Nursing: A Practical Approach,* 2nd edition. Burlington: Jones and Bartlett Learning.

Heidegger M (1976) [1954] *What Is Called Thinking?* London: Harper Perennial Reprint Edition.

Hempel C G (1945) Studies in the logic of confirmation (I). *Mind: A Quarterly Review of Psychology and Philosophy.* 213, 1–26.

Henderson A and Jones J (2017) Developing and maintaining compassionate care in nursing. *Nursing Standard.* 32(4), 60–69.

Herman T (2016) Search Engines and Ethics. *The Stanford Encyclopedia of Philosophy.* Zalta E N (ed.). Fall 2016 edition. Available online: https://plato.stanford.edu/entries/ethics-search/#Web20Era2000 (accessed 12.09.18).

Hicks D (2014). A new direction for science and values. *Synthese.* 191(14), 3271–3295. Available online: https://philpapers.org/rec/HICAND (accessed 20.12.18).

Hitchcock C (2004) Introduction: What is the Philosophy of Science? In Hitchcock C (ed.) *Contemporary Debates in Philosophy of Science,* pp. 1–19. Oxford: Blackwell Publishing.

Hohmann E, Brand J C, Rossi M J, and Lubowitz J H (2018) Expert Opinion is Necessary: Delphi Panel Methodology Facilitates a Scientific Approach to Consensus. *Arthroscopy.* 34(2), 349–351.

Holloway S (2017) The impact of postgraduate studies in wound healing on professional practice and personal development. *Wounds UK.* 13(3), 44–51.

Holmes D, Stuart J M, Perron A, and Geneviève R (2006) Deconstructing the evidence-based discourse in health sciences: truth, power and fascism. *International Journal of Evidence-Based Healthcare.* 4(3), 180–186.

Holmwood J (ed.) (2011) *A Manifesto for The Public University.* London: Bloomsbury Academic.

Holt-Ashley M (2000) Nurses pray: use of prayer and spirituality as a complimentary therapy in the intensive care setting. *AACN Clinical Issues: Advanced Practice in Acute and Critical Care.* 11(1), 60–67.

Hookway C (2013) *The Pragmatic Maxim: Essays on Peirce and Pragmatism.* Oxford: Oxford University Press.

Horgan T (2016) Mental Causation and Agency. Podcast produced by The School of Philosophy, Renmin University of China on 24.08.16. Available online: http://philo.ruc.edu.cn/ceap/ter ence-horgan-mental-causation-and-agency/ (accessed 12.04.18).

Hornsey M J, Harris E A, Bain P G, and Fielding K S (2016) Meta-analysis of the determinants and outcomes of belief in climate change. *Nature Climate Change.* 6, 622–626. Available online: www.na ture.com/articles/nclimate2943 (accessed 11.12.18).

Horsburgh D (2003) Evaluation of Qualitative Research. *Journal of Clinical Nursing.* 12(2), 307–312.

Hoyningen-Huene P (1987) Context Of Discovery And Context Of Justification. *Studies in History and Philosophy of Science: Part A.* 18(4), 501–515.

Hudis P and Anderson K B (eds) (2004) *The Rosa Luxemburg Reader.* New York: Monthly Review Press.

Hudson K, Duke G, Haas B, and Varnell G (2008) Navigating the evidence-based practice maze. *Journal of Nursing Management.* 16(4), 409–416.

Hughes E (2019) Inaugural Professorial Lecture of Professor Elizabeth Hughes: "Living Forever – A Dream or Reality?" University of Worcester. 20 March 2019.

Hutchison K J and Rogers W A (2012) Challenging the epistemological foundations of EBM: what kind of knowledge does clinical practice require? *Journal of Evaluation in Clinical Practice.* 18(5), 984–991.

Huxley A (2007) *Brave New World.* London: Vintage.

Huxley A (1937) *Ends and Means: An Enquiry into the Nature of Ideals and into the Methods Employed for their Realization.* London: Chatto & Windus.

Infantino L (1998) *Individualism in Modern Thought: From Adam Smith to Hayek.* London: Routledge.

Ingham-Broomfield R (2016) A nurses' guide to the hierarchy of research designs and evidence. *Journal of Advanced Nursing.* 33(3), 38–43.

Ioannidis J P A (2016) The Mass Production of Redundant, Misleading, and Conflicted Systematic Reviews and Meta-analyses. *The Milbank Quarterly.* 94(3), 485–514.

Issac J C (2015) For a More Public Political Science – From the editor. *Perspectives on Politics.* 13(2) 269–283.

Jacoby S F (2017) The insight and challenge of reflexive practice in an ethnographic study of black traumatically injured patients in Philadelphia. *Nursing Inquiry.* 24(3), 6.

Jain A (2016) The 5 Vs of Big Data – Healthcare Data Analytics – Blogpost. Available online: www. ibm.com/blogs/watson-health/the-5-vs-of-big-data/ (accessed 22.01.19).

James W (1912) *The Will to Believe: and Other Essays in Popular Philosophy, and Human Immortality.* Unknown (CreateSpace): Pantianos Classics Edition.

Janardhana N, Raghevendra G, Naidu D M, Prasanna L, and Chenappa T (2018) Caregiver Perspective and Understanding On road to Recovery. *Journal of Psychosocial Rehabilitation and Mental Health.* 5(1), 43–51.

Jernigan D K, Wadiak W, and Wang W M (eds) (2019) *Narrating Death: The Limit of Literature.* London: Routledge.

Joas H (1993) *Pragmatism and Social Theory.* Chicago: University of Chicago Press.

Jones-Schenk J, Leafman J, Wallace L, and Allen P (2017) Addressing the Cost, Value, and Student Debt in Nurse Education. *Nursing Economics.* 35(1), 7–29.

Johnson G, Pickup M, De Rooij E, and Léger R (2017) Research Openness in Canadian Political Science: Toward an Inclusive and Differentiated Discussion. *Canadian Journal of Political Science.* 50(1), 311–328.

Jung C G (2001) [1933] *Modern Man in Search of a Soul.* Translation: Dell W S and Baynes C F. London: Routledge.

Kahan D M (2013) Ideology, Motivated Reasoning, and Cognitive Reflection. *Judgment and Decision Making* 8(4), 407–424.

Kahneman D (2012) *Thinking, Fast and Slow*. London: Penguin Books.

Kanterian E (2015) Philosophy's Divide – Minerva podcast with Joshua Gottlieb on the relation between analytic and continental philosophy, August 2015. Available online: www.minerva-podcast. com/search/Kanterian (accessed 03.01.19).

Karcher S, Kirilova D, and Weber N (2016) Beyond the matrix: Repository services for qualitative data. *IFLA Journal*. 42(4), 292–302.

Kaya H, Işik B, Şenyüva E, and Kaya N (2017) Personal and professional values held by baccalaureate nursing students. *Nursing Ethics*. 24(6), 716–731.

Kayoko T and Atsushi A (2014) Analysis of 'care' and 'justice' involved in moral reasoning of nurse based on the Gilligan theory: A literature review using the Gilligan's protocol. *Open Journal of Nursing*. 4(2), 101–109.

Keenan G (2014). Big Data in Health Care: An Urgent Mandate to CHANGE Nursing EHRs! *Online Journal of Nursing Informatics*. 18(1). Available online: http://web.a.ebscohost.com.proxy.worc.ac.uk/ ehost/pdfviewer/pdfviewer?vid=8&sid=4dcf36db-fd78-44a3-8992-28c304592434%40sessionm gr4007 (accessed 04.02.19).

Keller P A and Block L G (1999) The effect of affect-based dissonance versus cognition-based dissonance on motivated reasoning and health-related persuasion. *Journal of Experimental Psychology: Applied*. 5(3), 302–313

Kerry R (2017) Why evidence-based healthcare has lost its way. *The Conversation*. Posted 31.10.17. Available online: https://theconversation.com/uk/health (accessed 01.01.19).

Keynes G (ed.) (1980) [1802] *The Letters of William Blake: With Related Documents*, 3rd edition. Oxford: Oxford University Press.

Khodabux R (2016) Identifying and defining research questions. *Nursing Times*. 112(3/4), 16–19.

King G, Schneer B, and White A (2017) How the news media activate expression and influence national agendas. *Science*. 358(6364), 776–780.

Kirman J (2016) Behavioural interviewing as part of values-based recruitment for postgraduate community nursing programmes. *Community Practitioner*. 89(8), 42–47.

Klein P D (2012) Infinitism and the Epistemic Regress Problem. In Tolksdorf S (ed.) *Conceptions of Knowledge*, pp. 487–508. Berlin: Walter de Gruyter.

Klein P D (2005) Infinitism Is the Solution to the Regress Problem. In Steup M and Sosa E (eds) *Contemporary Debates in Epistemology*, pp. 131–139. Oxford: Blackwell.

Klein R (1995) *The New Politics Of The NHS*, 3rd edition. Harlow: Longman Group Limited.

Kohn L T, Corrigan J M, and Donaldson M S (eds) (1999) *To Err Is Human: Building a Safer Health System*. Washington, DC: National Academies Press. Available online: www.nap.edu/read/9728/ chapter/1 (accessed 24.12.18).

Krauss A (2018) Why all randomised controlled trials produce biased results. *Annals of Medicine*. 50(4), 312–322.

Kriegbaum M, Liisberg K B, and Wallach-Kildemoes H (2017) Pattern if statin use changes following media coverage of its side effects. *Patient Preference and Adherence*. 11, 1151–1157.

Krips H (2010) The Politics of the Gaze: Foucault, Lacan and Žižek. *Culture Unbound (Journal of Current Cultural Research)*. 2, 91–102

Krislov M (2017) The Life-Shaping Power of Higher Education. Inside Higher Education. Available online: www.insidehighered.com/views/2017/10/06/importance-liberal-arts-transforming-lives-essay (accessed 09.10.18).

Krok-Schoen J L, Bernardo B M, Weier R C, Peng J, Katz M L, Reiter P L, Richardson M S, Pennell M L, Tatum C M, and Paskett E D (2018) Belief About Mandatory School Vaccinations and Vaccination Refusal Among Ohio Appalachian Parents: Do Demographic and Religious Factors, General Health, and Political Affiliation Play a Role? *The Journal of Rural Health*. 34(3), 283–292.

Kuhn D (2010) Teaching and learning science as argument. *Science Education*. 94(5), 810–824.

Kuhn D (1993) Science as argument: Implications for teaching and learning scientific thinking. *Science Education.* 77(3), 319–337.

Kuhn T S (1970) *The Structure of Scientific Revolutions,* 2nd edition – enlarged. Chicago: University of Chicago Press.

Kumsa M K, Chambon A, Yan M C, and Maiter S (2015) Catching the shimmers of the social: from the limits of reflexivity to methodological creativity. *Qualitative Research.* 15(4), 419–436.

Kunda Z (1990) The case for motivated reasoning. *Psychological Bulletin.* 108(3), 480–498.

Kurt A, Semler L, Meyers M, Porter B G, Jacoby J L, and Stello B (2017) Research Professionals' Perspectives, Barriers and Recommendations Regarding Minority Participation in Clinical Trials. *Journal of Racial and Ethnic Health Disparities.* 4(6), 1166–1174.

Kutney-Lee A, Sloane D M, and Aiken L H (2013) An Increase In The Number Of Nurses With Baccalaureate Degree Is Linked To Lower Rates Of Postsurgery Mortality. *Health Affairs.* 32(3), 579–586.

Lacan J (1998) *The Four Fundamental Concepts of Psycho-Analysis. The Seminar of Jacques Lacan – Book XI.* Miller J A (ed.). Translation Sheridan A. New York: W W Norton.

Lamiell J T (1998) 'Nomothetic' and 'Idiographic': Contrasting Windelband's Understanding with Contemporary Usage. *Theory and Psychology.* 8(1), 23–38.

Lang T (2004) Twenty Statistical Errors Even YOU Can Find In Biomedical Research Articles. *Croatian Medical Journal.* 45(4), 361–370.

Larden C (2017) "Imbalanced Energy Field" approved as a nursing diagnosis. *Healing Connection.* Available online: www.myhealingconnection.com/node/31 (accessed 22.02.19).

Latimer J and Gómez D L (2019) Intimate Entanglements: Affects, more-than-human intimacies and the politics of relations in science and technology. *The Sociological Review.* 67(2), 247–263.

Latour B and Woolgar S (1986) [1979] *Laboratory Life: The Construction of Scientific Facts.* Princeton: Princeton University Press.

Latzko-Toth G, Bonneau C, and Millette M (2017) Small Data, Thick Data: Thickening Strategies for Trace-Based Social Media Research. In Sloan L and Quan-Haase A (eds) *The SAGE Handbook of Social Media Research Methods,* pp. 119–214. London: SAGE.

Lau S R and Traulsen J M (2017) Are we ready to accept the challenge? Addressing the shortcomings of contemporary qualitative health research. *Research is Social and Administrative Pharmacy.* 13(2), 332–338.

Lavin M A, Meyer G, Krieger M, McNary P, Carlson J, Perry A, James D, and Civitan T (2002) Viewpoint: Essential differences between evidence-based nursing and evidence-based medicine. *International Journal of Nursing Terminologies and Classifications.* 13(3), 101–106.

Leary A (2017) What is a nurse? Baffling number of job roles leaves patients and bosses confused. *The Guardian,* 08.11.17. Available online: www.theguardian.com/healthcare-network/2017/nov/08/what-nurse-baffling-number-job-roles-leaves-patients-bosses-confused (accessed 14.11.18).

Lee A S and Baskerville R L (2012) Conceptualizing Generalizability: New Contribution and a Reply. *Management Information Systems Quarterly.* 36(3), 749–761.

Lee A S and Baskerville R L (2003) Generalizing Generalizability in Information Systems Research. *Information Systems Research.* 14(3), 221–243.

Lee I (2017) Big data: Dimensions, evolution, impacts, and challenges. *Business Horizons.* 60(3), 293–303.

LeLorier J, Grégoire G, Benhaddad A, Lapierre J, and Derderian F (1997) Discrepancies Between Meta-Analyses And Subsequent Large Randomized Controlled Trials. *The New England Journal of Medicine.* 337(8), 536–542.

Leung L (2015) Validity, reliability, and generalizability in qualitative research. *Journal of Family Medicine and Primary Care.* 4(3), 324–327.

Lewis J and Ritchie J (2003) Generalising from Qualitative Research. In Ritchie J and Lewis J (eds) (2003) *Qualitative Research Practice: A Guide for Social Science Students and Researchers,* pp. 263–286. London: Sage.

Liberati A, Altman D G, Tetzlaff J, Mulrow C, Gøtzsche P C, Ioannidis J P A, Clarke M, Devereaux P J, Kleijnen J, and Moher D (2009) The PRISMA Statement for Reporting Systematic Reviews and Meta-Analyses of Studies That Evaluate Health Care Interventions: Exploration and Elaboration. *Plos*

Medicine. 6(7). Available online: http://journals.plos.org/plosmedicine/article?id=10.1371/journal.pm ed.1000100 (accessed 08.12.18).

Lipp A and Fothergill A (2015) A guide to critiquing a research paper. Methodological appraisal of a paper on nurses in abortion care. *Nurse Education Today.* 35(3), e14–e17.

Lipscomb M (2017a) Introduction. In Lipscomb M (ed.) *Social Theory and Nursing*, pp. 1–9. London: Routledge.

Lipscomb M (2017b) Invited commentary – Nursing values: Divided we stand. *Nursing Inquiry.* 24(3), 3.

Lipscomb M (2016a) Introduction. In Lipscomb M (ed.) *Exploring Evidence-Based Practice: Debates and Challenges in Nursing*, pp. 1–10. London: Routledge.

Lipscomb M (2016b) Research appraisal and individual responsibility. In Lipscomb M (ed.) *Exploring Evidence-Based Practice: Debates and Challenges in Nursing*, pp. 165–179. London: Routledge.

Lipscomb M (2014a) *A Hospice in Change: Applied Social Realist Theory.* London: Routledge.

Lipscomb M (2014b) Research report appraisal: how much understanding is enough? *Nursing Philosophy.* 15(3), 157–170.

Lipscomb M (2012a) Abductive reasoning and qualitative research. *Nursing Philosophy.* 13(4), 244–256.

Lipscomb M (2012b) Questioning the use value of qualitative research findings. *Nursing Philosophy.* 13(2), 112–125.

Lipscomb M (2011) Challenging the Coherence of Social Justice as a Shared Nursing Value. *Nursing Philosophy.* 12(1), 4–11.

List C and Pettit P (2011) *Group Agency: The Possibility, Design, and Status of Corporate Agents.* Oxford: Oxford University Press.

Lockwood C (2015) Qualitative research synthesis: methodological guidance for systematic reviewers utilizing meta-aggregation. *International Journal of Evidence Based Healthcare.* 13(3), 179–187.

Long J W (2018) *Two Existential Theories of Knowledge: Epistemic Pragmatism And Contextualism.* Bloomington: iUniverse.

Lowenthal M M (2019) *Intelligence: From Secrets to Policy.* 8th edition. London: CQ Press - Sage.

Luchins A S (1942) Mechanisms in problem solving: The effect of Einstellung. *Psychological Monographs.* 54(6), 1–95. Available online: http://psycnet.apa.org/record/2011-21639-001 (accessed 13.12.18).

Lupia A and Elman C (2014) Openness in Political Science: Data Access and Research Transparency: Introduction. *Political Science and Politics.* 47(1), 19–42.

Lynch M P (2012) *In Praise of Reason.* Cambridge, MA: MIT Press.

Lyotard J-F (1984) [1979] *The Postmodern Condition: A Report on Knowledge.* Translation by Bennington G and Massumi B. Manchester: Manchester University Press.

Macfarlane B (2017) The REF is wrong: books are not inferior to papers. *Times Higher Education.* Available online: www.timeshighereducation.com/opinion/ref-wrong-books-are-not-inferior-papers (accessed 24.12.18).

Mackey A and Bassendowski S (2017) The History of Evidence-Based Practice in Nursing Education and Practice. *Journal of Professional Nursing.* 33(1), 51–55.

Macleod C and Nhamo-Murire M (2016) The emancipatory potential of nursing practice in relation to sexuality: a systematic literature review of nursing research 2009–2014. *Nursing Inquiry.* 23(3), 253–266.

Makary M and Daniel M (2016) Medical error – the third leading cause of death in the US. *British Medical Journal.* 353. Available online: www.bmj.com/content/bmj/353/bmj.i2139.full.pdf (accessed 06.02.19).

Maksimainen H (2017) Improving the Quality of Health Journalism: When Reliability meets Engagement. Reuters Institute Fellowship Paper. Reuters Institute for the Study of Journalism. University of Oxford. Available online: https://reutersinstitute.politics.ox.ac.uk/sites/default/files/2017-09/Maksimainen,%20Improving%20the%20Quality%20of%20Health%20Journalism_0.pdf (accessed 01.01.19).

Malterud K (2001) Qualitative research: standards, challenges, and guidelines. *The Lancet.* 358(9280), 483–488.

Mays M Z and Melnyk B M (2009) Guest Editorial: A Call for the Reporting of Effect Sizes in Research Reports to Enhance Critical Appraisal and Evidence-Based Practice. *World Views on Evidence-Based Nursing.* 6(3), 125–129.

Mazhindu D M, Griffiths L, Pook C, Erskine A, Ellis R, and Smith F (2016) The nurse match instrument: Exploring professional nursing identity and professional nursing values for future nurse recruitment. *Nurse Education in Practice.* 18(3), 36–45.

McCright A M, Dunlap R E, and Marquart-Pyatt S T (2016) Political ideology and views about climate change in the European Union. *Environmental Politics.* 25(2), 338–358.

McCullough M (2018) 'Abortion pill reversal' controversy heats up with new study – Blog post. *The Inquirer.* Daily News Phility.com. Posted 06.04.18. Available online: www.philly.com/philly/hea lth/abortion-pill-reversal-controversy-heats-up-with-new-study-20180406.html (accessed 26.02.19).

McMaster University (2019) Resources for Evidence-Based Practice: The 6S Pyramid. Health Sciences Library: Guides and Tutorials. McMaster University. Online resource updated 28.02.19. Available online: https://hslmcmaster.libguides.com/ebm (accessed 18.03.19).

McNamara M S (2005) Knowing and doing phenomenology: the implications of the critique of 'nursing phenomenology' for a phenomenological inquiry: a discussion paper. *International Journal of Nursing Studies.* 42(6), 695–704.

Mercier H and Sperber D (2018) *The Enigma of Reason: A New Theory of Human Understanding.* St Ives: Penguin Books.

Merton R K (1995) The Thomas Theorem and the Matthew Effect. *Social Forces.* 74(2), 379–422.

Merton R K (1948) The Self-Fulfilling Prophecy. *The Antioch Review.* 8(2), 193–210.

Methley A M, Campbell S, Chew-Graham C, McNally R, and Cheraghi-Sohi S (2014) PICO, PICOS and SPIDER: a comparison study of specificity and sensitivity in three search tools for qualitative systematic reviews. *BMC Health Services Research.* 14, 579. Available online: www.ncbi.nlm.nih. gov/pmc/articles/PMC4310146/ (accessed 11.10.18).

Mieronkoski R, Azimi I, Rahmani A M, Aantaa R, Terävä V, Liljeberg P, and Salanterä S (2017). The Internet of Things for Basic Nursing Care – A Scoping Review. *International Journal of Nursing Studies.* 69, 78–90.

Miers M (2016) Intra- and interprofessional working: Pitfalls and potential. In Lipscomb M (ed.) *Exploring Evidence-Based Practice: Debates and Challenges in Nursing,* pp. 29–43. London: Routledge.

Miers M (2000) Qualitative Research and the Generalizability Question: Standing Firm with Proteus. *The Qualitative Report.* 4(3). Available online: http://nsuworks.nova.edu/tqr/vol4/iss3/9/?utm_source=nsu works.nova.edu%2Ftqr%2Fvol4%2Fiss3%2F9&utm_medium=PDF&utm_campaign=PDFCoverPages (accessed 11.11.18).

Miles B M and Huberman A M (1994) *Qualitative Data Analysis,* 2nd edition. London: Sage.

Miller S L (2015) Values-based recruitment in health care. *Nursing Standard.* 29(21), 37–41.

Mills J and Hallinan C (2009) The social world of Australian practice nurses and the influence of medical dominance: an analysis of the literature. *International Journal of Nursing Practice.* 15(6), 489–494.

Milton C L (2017) The Ethics of Big Data and Nursing Science. *Nursing Science Quarterly.* 30(4), 300–302.

Mitchell G J, Pilkington B, Jonas-Simpson C M, Daiski I, Cross N L, Johnston N, O'Grady C P, Peisachovich E H, and Tang S Y (2016) Nursing education and complexity pedagogy: Faculty experiences with an e-learning platform. *Journal of Nursing Education and Practice.* 6(5), 60–68.

Mitchell K M and Clark A M (2018) Editorial: Five Steps to Writing More Engaging Qualitative Research. *International Journal of Qualitative Methodology.* 17(1), 1–3.

Mohammed M A, Moles R J, and Chen T F (2016) Meta-synthesis of qualitative research: the challenges and opportunities. *International Journal of Clinical Pharmacy.* 38(3), 695–704.

Moore A (2017) *Critical Elitism: Deliberation, Democracy, and the Problem of Expertise (Theories of Institutional Design).* Cambridge: Cambridge University Press.

Moravcsik A (2014a) Transparency: The revolution in qualitative research. *Political Science and Politics.* 47(1), 48–53.

Moravcsik A (2014b) Trust, but Verify: The Transparency Revolution and Qualitative International Relations. *Security Studies.* 23(4), 663–688.

Moravcsik A (2010) Active Citation: A Precondition for Replicable Qualitative Research. *Political Science and Politics.* 43(1), 29–35.

Morse J M (2015) Critical Analysis of Strategies for Determining Rigor in Qualitative Inquiry. *Qualitative Health Research.* 25(9), 1212–1222.

Morse J M, Barrett M, and Mayan M (2002) Verification Strategies for Establishing Reliability and Validity in Qualitative Research. *International Journal of Qualitative Methods.* 1(2), 13–22.

Moule P (2018) *Making Sense Of Research In Nursing, Health and Social Care,* 6th edition. London: Sage.

Murad M H, Asi N, Alsawas M, and Alahdab F (2016) New evidence pyramid. *Evidence Based Medicine.* 21(4). Available online: http://ebm.bmj.com/content/21/4/125 (accessed 08.12.18).

Murphy J, Goossen W, and Weber P (2017) Front Matter. In Murphy J, Goossen W and Weber P (eds) *Forecasting Informatics Competencies for Nurses in the Future of Connected Health – Studies in Health Technology and Informatics.* 232, pp. i–ix. Available online: http://ebooks.iospress.nl/volume/forecasting-informatics-competencies-for-nurses-in-the-future-of-connected-health-proceedings-of-the-nursing-informatics-post-conference-2016 (accessed 05.02.19).

Murray M (2018) The pre-history of health psychology in the United Kingdom: From natural science and psychoanalysis to social science, social cognition and beyond. *Journal of Health Psychology.* 23(3), 472–491.

MyoungJin K and Hayat M J (2015) Statistical Preparedness of Master's Degree-Prepared Nurses in the Workplace. *Nurse Educator.* 40(3), 144–147.

Nabi R L and Prestin A (2016) Unrealistic Hope and Unnecessary Fear: Exploring How Sensationalistic News Stories Influence Health Behavior Motivation. *Health Communication.* 31(9), 1115–1126.

Narayanasamy A and Narayanasamy M (2008) The healing power of prayer and its implications for nursing. *British Journal of Nursing.* 17(6), 394–398.

Nash K (2019) Neo-liberalisation, universities and the values of bureaucracy. *The Sociological Review.* 67(1), 178–193.

Neill C (2017) Writing a literature review. *Radiation Therapist.* 26(1), 89–91.

Nelson C D (2005) Crafting researcher subjectivity in ways that enact theory. *Journal of Language, Identity and Education.* 4(4), 315–320.

Nelson L D, Simmons J, and Simonsohn U (2018) Psychology's Renaissance. *Annual Review of Psychology.* 69(1), 511–534.

Nevo I and Slonim-Nevo V (2011) The Myth of Evidence-Based Practice: Towards Evidence-Informed Practice. *The British Journal of Social Work.* 41(6), 1176–1197.

Newell R and Burnard P (2006) *Research for Evidence-Based Practice: Vital Notes for Nurses.* Oxford: Blackwell.

Newton P, Chandler V, Morris-Thomson T, Sayer J, and Burke L (2015) Exploring selection and recruitment processes for newly qualified nurses: a sequential-explanatory mixed-method study. *Journal of Advanced Nursing.* 71(1), 54–64.

Niaz M (2007) Can Findings of Qualitative Research in Education be Generalised? *Quality and Quantity.* 41(3), 429–445.

Nietzsche F (2013) *On the Genealogy of Morals.* London: Penguin Classics.

Nilson C (2017) A Journey Towards Cultural Competence. *Journal of Transcultural Nursing.* 28(2), 119–127.

Nisbett R E and Wilson T D (1977). Telling more than we can know: Verbal reports on mental processes. *Psychological Review,* 84(3), 231–259.

NMC – Nursing and Midwifery Council (2018) The Code: Professional standards of practice and behaviour for nurses and midwives. Available online: www.nmc.org.uk/standards/code/ (accessed 19.12.18).

Noblit G W and Hare R D (1988) *Meta-Ethnography, Synthesising Qualitative Studies.* London: Sage.

Nolfi D A, Lockhart J S, and Myers C R (2015) Predatory Publishing: What You Don't Know Can Hurt You. *Nurse Educator.* 40(5), 217–219.

Nordestgaard B G (2018) Why do the media report negative news about statins? *European Heart Journal.* 39(5), 337–338.

Norlyk A, Haahr A, Dreyer P, and Martinsen B (2017) Lost in transformation? Reviving ethics of care in hospital cultures of evidence-based healthcare. *Nursing Inquiry*. 24(3), n/a-n/a. 7p.

Northwood M, Ploeg J, Markle-Reid M, and Sherifali D (2018) Integrative review of the social determinants of health in older adults with multimorbidity. *Journal of Advanced Nursing*. 74(1), 45–60.

Nozick R (1974) *Anarchy, State, and Utopia*. New York: Basic Books.

Nuzzo R (2014) Statistical Errors: P values, the 'gold standard' of statistical validity, are not as reliable as many scientists assume. *Nature*. 506, 150–152.

Oakeshott M (1991) [1947] Rationalism in politics. In *Rationalism in Politics and Other Essays*, pp. 5–42. Indianapolis: Liberty-Press.

O'Conner S (2018) Big Data and Data Science in Healthcare: What Nurses and Midwifes Need to Know. *Journal of Clinical Nursing*. 27(15–16), 2921–2922.

Oermann M H, Conklin J L, Nicoll L H, Chinn P L, Ashton K S, Edie A H, Amarasekara S, and Budinger S C (2016) Study of Predatory Open Access Nursing Journals. *Journal of Nursing Scholarship*. 48(6), 624–632.

Ofri D (2019) Perchance to Think – Perspective. *The New England Journal of Medicine*. 380(13), 1197–1199.

O'Grady J, Roche M, Brady A-M, and Prizeman G (2017) Core values of nursing care. *World of Irish Nursing and Midwifery*. 25(1), 47.

O'Sullivan E D and Schofield S J (2018) Cognitive bias in clinical medicine. *Journal of Royal College of Physicians of Edinburgh*. 48(3), 225–232.

Paley J (2017) *Phenomenology as Qualitative Research: A Critical Analysis of Meaning Attribution*. London: Routledge.

Paley J (2016) Evidence and the qualitative research analogous structure. In Lipscomb M (ed.) *Exploring Evidence-Based Practice: Debates and Challenges in Nursing*, pp. 132–150. London: Routledge.

Parahoo K (2006) *Nursing Research: Principles, Process and Issues*, 2nd edition. Basingstoke: Palgrave Macmillan.

Parkhurst J (2017) *The Politics of Evidence: From Evidence-Based Policy to the Good Governance of Evidence*. London: Routledge.

Parse R R (2017) Seeing Beyond the At-Hand. *Nursing Science Quarterly*. 30(3), 193.

Parse R R (2016) Where Have All the Nursing Theories Gone? *Nursing Science Quarterly*. 29(2), 101–102.

Parse R R, Barrett E A M, Bourgeois M, Dee V, Egan E, Germain C, King I, Koerner J, Neuman B, Newman M, Roy C, Walker L, Watson J, and Wolf G. (2000). Nursing theory-guided practice: A definition. *Nursing Science Quarterly*. 13(2), 177.

Patterson F, Prescott-Clements L, Zibarras L, Edwards H, Kerrin M, and Cousans F (2016) Recruiting for values in healthcare: a preliminary review of the evidence. *Advances in Health Sciences Education*. 21(4), 859–881.

Pawson R (2006) *Evidence-based Policy: A Realist Perspective*. London: Sage.

Peirce C P (1877) The Fixation of Belief. *Popular Science Monthly*. 12, 1–15. Available online: www.bocc.ubi.pt/pag/peirce-charles-fixation-belief.pdf (accessed 04.01.18).

Perin C (2010) *The Demands of Reason: An Essay on Pyrrhonian Scepticism*. Oxford: Oxford University Press.

Perry B (2005) The power of the simplest gesture: prayer, music, touch, and silence can all be therapeutic in caring for the seriously ill. *Health Progress*. 86(5), 50–53.

Perry C, Henderson A, and Grealish L (2018) The behaviours of nurses that increase student accountability for learning in clinical practice: An integrative review. *Nurse Education Today*. 65, 177–186.

Petrovskaya O (2014) Is there nursing phenomenology after Paley? Essay on rigorous reading. *Nursing Philosophy*. 15(1), 60–71.

Petrovskaya O, McDonald C, and McIntyre M (2011) Dialectic of the university: a critique of instrumental reason in graduate nursing education. *Nursing Philosophy*. 12(4), 239–247.

Phillips J R (2017) New Rogerian Theoretical Thinking About Unitary Science. *Nursing Science Quarterly*. 30(3), 223–226.

Plato (2007) *The Republic*. Translation, D. Lees. London: Penguin Classics.

Playle J F (1995) Humanism and positivism in nursing: contradictions and conflicts. *Journal of Advanced Nursing.* 22(5), 979–984.

Polit D F and Beck C T (2010) Generalization in quantitative and qualitative research: Myths and strategies. *International Journal of Nursing Studies.* 47(11), 1451–1458.

Polo A J, Makol B A, Castro A S, Colón-Quintana N, Wagstaff A E, and Guo S (2019) Diversity in randomised controlled trials of depression: A 36-year review. *Clinical Psychology Review.* 67, 22–35.

Powell M B and Wright R (2008) Investigative Interviewers' Perceptions of the Value of Different Training Tasks on their Adherence to Open-Ended Questions with Children. *Journal of Psychiatry, Phycology and Law.* 15(2), 272–283.

Pradeu T (2017) Lakatos Award Lecture – Podcast. The London School of Economics and Political Science. Available online: www.lse.ac.uk/website-archive/newsAndMedia/videoAndAudio/cha nnels/publicLecturesAndEvents/player.aspx?id=3931 (accessed 07.02.19).

Price H H (1967) Some Considerations About Belief. In Griffiths A P (ed.) *Knowledge And Belief,* pp. 41–59. Oxford: Oxford University Press. Originally published in: *Proceedings of the Aristotelian Society (1934-1935).* 35, 229–252.

Pritchard D (2019) *Epistemic Angst: Radical Skepticism and the Groundlessness of Our Believing,* reprint edition. Woodstock: Princetown University Press in association with Soochow University.

Probyn J, Howarth M, and Maz J (2016) The 'middle bit': how to appraise qualitative research. *British Journal of Cardiac Nursing.* 11(5), 248–254.

Punch K F (2005) *Introduction to Social Research: Quantitative and Qualitative Approaches,* 2nd edition. London: Sage.

Rafferty A M (2018) Nurses as change agents for a better future in health care: the politics of drift and dilution. *Health Economics, Policy and Law.* 13(3–4), 475–491.

Rafferty A M (1995) Art, science and social science in nursing: occupational origins and disciplinary integrity. *Nursing Inquiry.* 2(3), 141–148.

Rand A (1996) *Atlas Shrugged.* New York: Signet-New American Library, Penguin (USA).

Rand A (1984a) [1971] Don't let it go. In *Philosophy: Who Needs It?* pp. 205–215. New York: Signet Books.

Rand A (1984b) [1972] Fairness Doctrine for Education. In *Philosophy: Who Needs It?* pp. 189–198. New York: Signet Books.

Rand A (1964) *The Virtue of Selfishness: A New Concept of Egoism.* Harmondsworth: Penguin Books.

Rasmussen L M and Montgomery P (2018) The prevalence of and factors associated with inclusion of non-English language studies in Campbell systematic reviews: a survey and meta-epidemiological study. *BMC.* 7, 129. Available online: https://systematicreviewsjournal.biomedcentral.com/articles/ 10.1186/s13643-018-0786-6 (accessed 10.11.18).

Rasmussen P, Henderson A, Andrew N, and Conroy T (2018) Factors Influencing Registered Nurses' Perceptions of Their Professional Identity: An Integrative Literature Review. *The Journal of Continuing Education in Nursing.* 49(5), 225–232.

Rawls J (1971) *A Theory of Justice.* Oxford: Oxford University Press.

Redlawsk D P (2002) Hot Cognition or Cool Consideration? Testing the Effects of Motivated Reasoning on Political Decision Making. *The Journal of Politics.* 64(4), 1021–1044.

Rescher N (2000) *Realistic Pragmatism: An Introduction to Pragmatic Philosophy.* Albany: State University of New York Press.

Rescher N (1999) *The Limits of Science,* revised edition. Pittsburgh: University of Pittsburgh Press.

Ricoeur P (2007) *Evil: A Challenge to Philosophy And Theology.* Translation: Bowden J. London: Continuum.

Ringham C (2012) Narratives and Embodied Knowledge in the NICU. *Neonatal Network.* 31(1), 16–19.

Risling T (2017) Issues for Debate – Educating the nurses of 2025: Technology trends of the next decade. *Nurse Education in Practice.* 22, 89–92.

Risjord M (2010) *Nursing Knowledge: Science, Practice, and Philosophy.* Oxford: Wiley Blackwell.

Risjord M W (2014) *Philosophy of Social Science: A Contemporary Introduction.* London: Routledge.

Robinson E, Bevelander K E, Field M, and Jones A (2018) Methodological and reporting quality in laboratory studies of human eating behaviour. Reprint. *Appetite*. 125, 486–491.

Rojas E, Munoz-Gama J, Sepúlveda M, and Capurro D (2016) Process mining in healthcare: a literature review. *Journal of Biomedical Informatics*. 61, 224–236.

Rolfe G (2016a) Evidence-based practice and practice-based evidence. In Lipscomb M (ed.) *Exploring Evidence-Based Practice: Debates and Challenges in Nursing*, pp. 99–112. London: Routledge.

Rolfe G (2016b) Exercising the nursing imagination: putting values and scholarship back into research. *Journal of Research in Nursing*. 21(7), 517–527.

Rolfe G (2015) Foundations for a human science of nursing: Gadamer, Laing, and the hermeneutics of caring. *Nursing Philosophy*. 16(3), 141–152.

Rolfe G (2012) *The University in Dissent: Scholarship in the Corporate University*. London: Routledge.

Rolfe G (2010) A reply to 'Why nursing has not embraced the clinician-scientist role' by Martha MacKay: nursing science and the postmodern menace. *Nursing Philosophy*. 11(2), 136–140.

Rolfe G (2005) The deconstructing angel: nursing, reflection and evidence-based practice. *Nursing Inquiry*. 12(2), 78–86.

Rolfe G, Segrott J, and Jordan S (2008) Tensions and contradictions in nurses' perspectives of evidence-based practice. *Journal of Nursing Management*. 16(4), 440–451.

Rose D (2017) Service user/survivor-led research in mental health: epistemological possibilities. *Disability and Society*. 32(6), 773–789.

Rose E (2013) *On Reflection: An Essay on Technology, Education, and the Status of Thought in the Twenty-First Century*. Toronto: Canadian Scholars Press.

Rose G (2011) [1995] *Love's Work: A Reckoning With Life*. New York: New York Review Books.

Rosenberg G R (2017) 9 Steps For Creating A Research Essay Or Literature Review Paper. Available online: www.linkedin.com/pulse/9-steps-creating-research-essay-literature-review-paper-rosenberg/ (accessed 02.10.17).

Rosser E (2016) Nursing history: From conformity to challenging practice. *British Journal of Nursing*. 25(22), 1270–1270.

Rosser E, Neal D, Reeve J, Valentine J, and Grey R (2016) Evidence-based practice as taught and experienced: Education, practice and context. In Lipscomb M (ed.) *Exploring Evidence-Based Practice: Debates and Challenges in Nursing*, pp. 44–60. London: Routledge.

Rothbard M (2016) [1971] Ludwig von Mises and the Paradigm of our age. In Salerno J T and McCaffrey M (eds) *The Rothbard Reader*, pp. 72–86. Auburn: Ludwig von Mises Institute.

Rothbard M (2009) *The Anatomy of the State*. Auburn: Ludwig von Mises Institute.

Rousseau D M and Tijoriwala S A (1999) What's a good reason to change? Motivated reasoning and social accounts in promoting organizational change. *Journal of Applied Psychology*. 84(4), 514–528.

Rowson K (2016) How to conduct a literature review: a process that should be familiar to nurses. *HIV Nursing*. 16(3), 92–93.

Royal College of Nursing (2002) *Witnessing Resuscitation: Guidance for Nursing Staff*. London: Royal College of Nursing.

Ryan G and Rutty J (2019) Philosophy and quality? TAPUPASM as an approach to rigour in critical realist research. *Nurse Researcher*. 27(1), 33–40.

Rycroft-Malone J, Seers K, Titchen A, Harvey G, Kitson A, and McCormack B (2004) What counts as evidence in evidence-based practice? *Journal of Advanced Nursing*. 47(1), 81–90.

Ryle G (1945) Knowing How And Knowing That. Presidential Address. Series: Papers read before the Society. The Aristotelian Society – University of London Club. November 5.

Saimbert M, Pierce J, and Hargwood P (2017) Developing Clinical Questions For Systematic Review. In Holly C, Salmond S, and Saimbert (eds) *Comprehensive Systematic Review for Advanced Practice Nursing*, 2nd edition, pp. 79–103. New York: Springer.

Sandwell M and Carson P (2005) Developing numeracy in child branch students. *Paediatric Nursing*. 17 (9), 24–26.

Salmon W C (2013) [1992] Scientific Explanation. In Bird A and Ladyman J (eds) *Arguing About Science*, pp. 337–365. London: Routledge. Originally in Salmon M E, Earman J, Glymour C, Lennox J G,

Machamer P, McGuire J E, Norton J D, Salmon W C, and Schaffner (eds) *Introduction to the Philosophy of Science: A Text by Members of the Department of the History and Philosophy of Science of the University of Pittsburgh.* Englewood Cliffs: Prentice-Hall.

Santangelo T, Novosel L C, Cook B G, and Gapsis M (2015) Using the 6S Pyramid to Identify Research-Based Instructional Practices for Students with Learning Disabilities. *Learning Disabilities: Research and Practice.* 30(2), 91–101.

Santiago-Delefosse M, Gavin A, Bruchez C, Roux P, and Stephen S L (2016) Quality of qualitative research in the health sciences: Analysis of the common criteria present in 58 assessment guidelines by expert users. *Social Science and Medicine.* 148, 142–151.

Sartre J P (1996) *Being and Nothingness: An Essay on Phenomenological Ontology.* London: Routledge.

Sarver W, Cichra N, and Kline M (2015) Perceived benefits, motivators, and barriers to Advancing Nurse education: removing barriers to improve success. *Nursing Education Perspectives.* 36(3), 153–156.

Saunders B, Sim J, Kingstone T, Baker S, Waterfield J, Bartlam B, Burroughs H, and Jinks C (2018) Saturation in qualitative research: exploring its conceptualization and operationalization. *Quality and Quantity: International Journal of Methodology.* 52(4), 1893–1907.

Saunders H and Vehviläinen-Julkunen K (2018) Key considerations for selecting instruments when evaluating healthcare professionals' evidence-based practice competencies: A discussion paper. *Journal of Advanced Nursing.* 74(10), 2301–2311.

Scammell J (2016) 'Prioritise people': the importance of anti-oppressive practice. *British Journal of Nursing.* 25(4), 226.

Scherer R W, Meerpohl J J, Pfeifer N, Schmucker C, Schwarzer G, and von Elm E (2018) Full publication of results initially presented in abstracts. Cochrane Database of Systematic Reviews. Issue 11 – Art No MR000005. Available online: www.cochranelibrary.com/cdsr/doi/10.1002/14651858. MR000005.pub4/full (accessed 26.02.19).

Schreiber C A, Creinin M D, Atrio J, Sonalkar S, Ratcliffe S J, and Barnhart K T (2018) Mifepristone Pretreatment for the Medical Management of Early Pregnancy Loss. *New England Journal of Medicine.* 378(23), 2161–2170.

Schryen, Wagner, and Benlian (2015) Theory of Knowledge for Literature Reviews: An Epistemological Model, Taxonomy and Empirical Analysis of IS Literature. Thirty Sixth International Conference on Information Systems. Fort Worth. Available online: https://epub.uni-regensburg.de/32455/1/Theory%20of%20Knowledge%20for%20IS%20Literature%20Reviews%20-%20Revised%20Version.pdf (accessed 20.12.18).

Schulenburg J (2015) Considerations for Complementary and Alternative Interventions for Pain. *AORN Journal.* 101(3), 319–326.

Schwartz-Shea P and Yanow D (2016) Legitimizing Political Science or Splitting the Discipline? Reflections on DA-RT and the Policy-making Role of a Professional Association. *Politics and Gender,* 12(3), 1–19.

Seale C (1999) *The Quality of Qualitative Research.* London: Sage.

Sellman D (2019) Editorial: On writers and their biases. *Nursing Philosophy.* 20(1), 1–2.

Sellman D (2016) The practice of nursing research: getting ready for 'ethics' and the matter of character. *Nursing Inquiry.* 23(1), 24–31.

Setia M S (2017) Methodology Series Module 10: Qualitative Health Research. *Indian Journal of Dermatology.* 62(4), 367–370.

Sethi T (2018) Big Data to Big Knowledge for Next Generation Medicine: A Data Science Roadmap. In Srinivasan S (ed.) *Guide to Big Data Applications: Studies in Big Data,* vol 26, pp. 371–399. Cham: Springer.

Shamseer L, Moher D, Maduekwe O, Turner L, Barbour V, Burch R, Clark J, Galipeau J, Roberts J, and Shea B J (2017) Potential predatory and legitimate biomedical journals: can you tell the difference? A cross-sectional comparison. *BMC Medicine.* Available online: http://web.a.ebscohost.com.proxy.worc.ac.uk/ehost/pdfviewer/pdfviewer?vid=5&sid=78902221-e71b-4903-be81-d77d484cd85e%40sessionmgr4008 (accessed 28.11.18).

Sharon D and Grinberg K (2018) Does the level of emotional intelligence affect the degree of success in nursing studies? *Nurse Education Today*. 64, 21–26.

Shatz D (1983) Foundationalism, Coherentism, and the Levels Gambit. *Synthese*. 55(1), 97–118.

Shen F, Sheer V C, and Li R (2015) Impact of Narratives on Persuasion in Health Communication: A Meta-Analysis. *Journal of Advertising*. 44(2), 105–113.

Shenton, A (2004) Strategies for ensuring trustworthiness in qualitative research projects. *Education for Information*. 22(2), 63–75.

Sher G (2016) *Epistemic Friction: An Essay on Knowledge, Truth, and Logic*. Oxford: Oxford University Press.

Shesterinina A, Pollack M A, and Arriola L R (2019) Evidence from Researcher Interactions with Human Participants. American Political Science Association. Available online: https://papers.ssrn.com/sol3/papers.cfm?abstract_id=3333392 (accessed 29.03.19).

Shields L, Morrall P, Goodman B, Purcell C, and Watson R (2012) Care to be a nurse? Reflections on a radio broadcast and its ramifications for nursing today. *Nurse Education Today*. 32(5), 614–617.

Shojania K G and Dixon-Woods M (2016) Estimating deaths due to medical error: the ongoing controversy and why it matters. *BMJ Quality and Safety*. 26(5). Available online: http://qualitysafety.bmj.com/content/26/5/423#ref-4 (accessed 21.12.18).

Siegel S (2017) *The Rationality of Perception*. Oxford: Oxford University Press.

Siegfried T (2018) Informed wisdom trumps rigid rules when it comes to medical evidence. *Science News*. Available online: www.sciencenews.org/blog/context/informed-wisdom-trumps-rigid-rules-when-it-comes-medical-evidence (accessed 12.12.18).

SIGN – The Scottish Intercollegiate Guidelines Network Hierarchy (2014) *SIGN 50: A Guideline Developer's Handbook*. Edinburgh: SIGN. Available online: www.sign.ac.uk/guidelines/fulltext/50/index.html (accessed 14.10.18).

Skela-Savič B, Hvalič-Touzery S, and Pesjak K (2017) Professional values and competencies as explanatory factors for the use of evidence-based practice in nursing. *Journal of Advanced Nursing*. 73(8), 1910–1923.

Sloman S and Fernbach P (2017) *The Knowledge Illusion: Why We Never Think Alone*. London: Macmillan.

Smaldino P E and McElreath R (2016) The natural selection of bad science. *Royal Society. Open Sci*. 3, 160384. Available online: http://rsos.royalsocietypublishing.org/content/3/9/160384 (accessed 10.02.19).

Smith A (2010) *The Theory of Moral Sentiments*. London: Penguin Classics.

Smith A B, Agar M, Delaney G, Descallar J, Dobell-Brown K, Grand M, Aung J, Patel P, Kaadan N, and Girgis A (2018) Lower trial participation by culturally and linguistically diverse (CALD) cancer patients is largely due to language barriers. *Asia-Pacific Journal of Clinical Oncology*. 14(1), 52–60.

Smith B (2018) Generalizability in qualitative research: misunderstandings, opportunities and recommendations for the sport and exercise sciences. *Qualitative Research in Sport, Exercise and Health*. 10(1), 137–149.

Snow C P (1960) *The Two Cultures and The Scientific Revolution*. The Rede Lecture 1959. Cambridge: The Syndics of The Cambridge University Press.

Springer R A and Clinton M E (2017) 'Philosophy Lost': Inquiring into the effects of the corporatized university and its implications for graduate nursing education. *Nursing Inquiry*. 24(4), e1–8.

Spry C and Mierzwinski-Urban M (2018) The impact of the peer review of literature search strategies in support of rapid review reports. *Research Synthesis Methods*. 9(4), 521–526.

SPUC – Society for the Protection of Unborn Children (2019) Homepage. Available online: www.spuc.org.uk/ (accessed 22.02.19).

Spurlock Jr D (2017) Beyond $p < .05$: Toward a Nightingalean Perspective on Statistical Significance for Nursing Education Researchers. *Journal of Nursing Education*. 56(8), 453–455.

Stanley S K, Wilson M S, and Milfont T L (2017) Exploring short-term longitudinal effects of right-wing authoritarianism and social dominance orientation on environmentalism. *Personality and Individual Differences*. 108, 174–177.

Staples J N, Lester J, Li A, Walsh C, Cass I, Karlan B Y, Bresee C, and Rimel B J (2018) Language as a barrier to clinical trial accrual: assessing consenting team knowledge and practices for cancer clinical trial consent among low English fluency patients. *BMC.* 38, 14. Available online: https://appliedcr.biomedcentral.com/articles/10.1186/s41241-018-0065-9 (accessed on 13.11.18).

Stark P B and Saltelli A (2018) Cargo-cult statistics and scientific crisis. Royal Statistical Society. *Significance.* 15(4), 40–43.

Stavrianopoulos T (2016) Impact of a Nurses-Led Telephone Intervention Program on the Quality of Life in Patients with Heart Failure in a District Hospital of Greece. *Health Science Journal.* 10(4), 1–8.

Stephenson J (2017) Exclusive: 'Our image is out of date', says nurse academic. *Nursing Times.* Available online: www.nursingtimes.net/news/education/exclusive-our-image-is-out-of-date-says-nurse-academic/7021953.article (accessed 15.11.18).

Stock K (2016) Interview: Philosophy Bites – Kathleen Stock on Fiction and the Emotions – Podcast. Available online: https://philosophybites.com/2016/11/kathleen-stock-on-fiction-and-the-emotions.html (accessed 20.01.19).

Stokes D (2012) Perceiving and desiring: a new look at the cognitive penetrability of experience. *Philosophical Studies.* 158(3), 477–492.

Strasak A M, Qamruz Z, Pfeiffer K P, Göbel G, and Ulmer H (2007) Statistical errors in medical research – a review of common pitfalls. *Swiss Medical Weekly.* 137(03–04), 44–49.

Sunstein C R (2015) *Choosing Not TO Choose: Understanding the Value of Choice.* Oxford: Oxford University Press.

Sutherland S (2013) *Irrationality: The Enemy Within.* London: Printer and Martin Ltd.

Swedberg R (2014) *The Art of Social Theory.* Woodstock: Princetown University Press.

Swinburne R (2001) *Epistemic Justification.* Oxford: Clarendon Press.

Synder J (2014) Active Citation: In Search of Smoking Guns or Meaningful Context? *Security Studies.* 23(4), 708–714.

Tanne J H (2018) Conflicts of interest pervade US treatment guidelines, reports say. *BMJ.* 363, k4543. Available online: www.bmj.com/content/363/bmj.k4543 (accessed 12.12.18).

Tanney J (2013) Interview: New Books Network – Philosophy. Discussing *Rules, Reasons and Self-Knowledge* – Podcast. Available online: https://newbooksnetwork.com/julia-tanney-rules-reasons-and-self-knowledge-harvard-up-2012/ (accessed 10.01.19).

Tapp D and Mireille L (2017) The Humanbecoming theory as a reinterpretation of the symbolic interactionism: a critique of its specific nature and scientific underpinnings. *Nursing Philosophy.* 18(2), 1–13.

Tetley J, Dobson F, Jack K, Pearson B, and Walker E (2016) Building a values based culture in nurse education. *Nurse Education in Practice.* 16(1), 152–155.

Tetlock P and Gardner D (2016) *Super-Forecasting: The Art and Science of Prediction.* London: Random House.

Tett G (2016) *The Silo Effect: Why Every Organisation Needs to Disrupt Itself to Survive.* London: Abacus.

Thaler R H and Sunstein C R (2009) *Nudge: Improving Decisions About Health, Wealth and Happiness.* London: Penguin Books.

Thomas C, Didierjean A, and Kuhn G (2018) It is magic! How impossible solutions prevent the discovery of obvious ones? *Quarterly Journal of Experimental Psychology.* 71(12), 2481–2487.

Thomas G (2011) *How to Do Your Case Study: A Guide for Students and Researchers.* London: Sage.

Thomas S J (2016) Does evidence-based healthcare have room for the self? *Journal of Evaluation in Clinical Practice.* 22(4), 502–508.

Thompson A (2002) *Critical Reasoning: A Practical Introduction,* 2nd edition. London: Routledge.

Thompson P (2017) Avoiding the laundry list literature review – Blogpost: Available online: https://patthomson.net/2017/09/11/avoiding-the-laundry-list-literature-review/ (accessed 20.02.19).

Thomson W (1889) Electrical Units of Measurement – A Lecture delivered at the Institution of Civil Engineers, May 3rd, 1883. In *Popular Lectures and Addresses,* vol 1: Constitution of Matter, pp. 73–136. London: MacMillan and Co.

Thorne S (2019) Editorial: On the Evolving World of What Constitutes Qualitative Synthesis. *Qualitative Health Research*. 29(1), 3–6.

Thorne S (2018a) Editorial: In search of our collective voice. *Nursing Inquiry*. 25(4), 1–3.

Thorne S (2018b) Editorial: Rediscovering the "narrative" review. *Nursing Inquiry*. 25(3), 1–2.

Thorne S (2017) Metasynthetic Madness: What kind of monster have we created? *Qualitative Health Research*. 27(1), 3–12.

Thorne S (2016a) *Interpretive Description: Qualitative Research for Applied Practice*. Second edition. London: Routledge.

Thorne S (2016b) The status and use value of qualitative research findings: New ways to make sense of qualitative work. In Lipscomb M (ed.) *Exploring Evidence-Based Practice: Debates and Challenges in Nursing*, pp. 151–164. London: Routledge.

Thorne S (2015) Does nursing represent a unique angle of vision? If so, what is it? *Nursing Inquiry*. 22(4), 283–284.

Thorne S, Jensen L, Kearney M H, Nobit G, and Sandelowski M (2004) Qualitative Metasynthesis: Reflections on Methodological Orientation and Ideological Agenda. *Qualitative Health Research*. 14(10), 1342–1365.

Topaz M and Pruinelli L (2017) Big Data and Nursing: Implications for the future. In Murphy J, Goossen W and Weber P (eds) *Forecasting Informatics Competencies for Nurses in the Future of Connected Health – Studies in Health Technology and Informatics*, 232, pp. 165–171. Available online: http://ebooks.iospress.nl/volume/forecasting-informatics-competencies-for-nurses-in-the-future-of-connected-health-proceedings-of-the-nursing-informatics-post-conference-2016 (accessed 05.10.18).

Tracy S J (2010) Qualitative quality: eight 'big-tent' criteria for excellent qualitative research. *Qualitative Inquiry*. 16(10), 835–851.

Traynor M (2013) *Nursing in Context: Policy, Politics, Profession*. Basingstoke: Palgrave Macmillan.

Trusted J (1987) *Moral Principles and Social Values*. London: Routledge and Kegan Paul.

Tsang E W K and Williams J N (2012) Generalization and induction: Misconceptions, clarifications and a classification of induction. *MIS Quarterly*. 36(3), 729–748.

Tubbs N (1998) What Is Love's Work? *Women: A Cultural Review*. 9(1), 34–46.

Tuckett A (2015) Speaking with one voice: A study of the values of new nursing graduates and the implications for educators. *Nurse Education in Practice*. 15(4), 258–264.

Van Deemter K (2010) *Not Exactly: In Praise of Vagueness*. Oxford: Oxford University Press.

van Rijnsoever F J (2016) (I Can't Get No) Saturation: A simulation and guidelines for sample sizes in qualitative research. *PLOS one*. Available online: http://journals.plos.org/plosone/article?id=10.1371/journal.pone.0181689 (accessed 17.12.18).

van Wijngaarden E, van der Meide H, and Dahlberg K (2017) Researching Health Care as a Meaningful Practice: Toward a Nondualistic View on Evidence for Qualitative Research. *Qualitative Health Research*. 27(11), 1738–1747.

Varpio L, Ajjawi R, Monrouxe L V, O'Brien B C, and Rees C E (2017) Shedding the cobra effect: problematising thematic emergence, triangulation, saturation and member checking. *Medical Education*. 51(1), 40–50.

von Mises L (1998) *Human Action: A Treatise on Economics*. Alabama: The Ludwig von Mises Institute.

Wangensteen S, Finnbakk E, Adolfsson A, Kristjansdottir G, Roodbol P, Ward H, and Fagerström L (2018) Postgraduate nurses' self-assessment of clinical competence and need for further training. A European cross-sectional survey. *Nurse Education Today*. 62, 101–106.

Warburton P, Sherrington S, Kirton J, Ryland I, and Jinks A (2010) An evaluation of an online numeracy assessment tool. *Nursing Standard*. 24(30), 62–68.

Ward PR, Attwell K, Meyer SB, Rokkas P, and Leask J (2017) Understanding the perceived logic of care by vaccine-hesitant and vaccine-refusing parents: A qualitative study in Australia. *PLoS ONE* 12(10). Available online: http://journals.plos.org/plosone/article?id=10.1371/journal.pone.0185955 (accessed 23.02.19).

Watkins L M (2015) Professionalism in Nursing. *Mississippi RN*. 77(2), 1.

Watson J (2018) *Unitary Caring Science: The Philosophy and Praxis of Nursing.* Louisville: University Press of Colorado.

Watson R (2016) You're more likely to survive hospital if your nurse has a degree – Blog. *The Conversation.* Available online: https://theconversation.com/amp/youre-more-likely-to-survive-hospital-if-your-nurse-has-a-degree-61838?__twitter_impression=trueq (accessed 02.01.19).

Weber M (2012) [1905] *The Protestant Ethic and The Spirit of Capitalism.* USA: Renaissance Classics.

Weissman D (1993) *Truth's Debt to Value.* New Haven: Yale University Press.

Welch C and Piekkari R (2017) How should we (not) judge the 'quality' of qualitative research? A reassessment of current evaluative criteria in International Business. *Journal of World Business.* 52(5), 714–725.

Welp A, Johnson A, Nguyen H, and Perry L (2018) The importance of reflecting on practice: How personal professional development activities affect perceived teamwork and performance. *Journal of Clinical Nursing.* Available online: https://doi.org/10.1111/jocn.14519 (accessed 18.09.18).

Werner P J (2018) Moral Perception without (Prior) Moral Knowledge. *Journal of Moral Philosophy.* 15(2), 164–181.

White H D, Boell S K, Yu H, Davis M, Concepción S W, and Cole F T H (2009) Libcitations: A Measure for Comparative Assessment of Book Publications in the Humanities and Social Sciences. *Journal of the American Society for Information Science and Technology.* 60(6), 1083–1096.

Whittemore R and Knafl K (2005) The integrative review: Updated methodology. *Journal of Advanced Nursing.* 52(5), 546–553.

Wieringa S, Engebretson E, Heggen K, and Greenhalgh T (2018) Rethinking bias and truth in evidence-based health care. *Journal of Evaluation in Clinical Practice.* 24(5), 930–938.

Wilson J C (1967) The Relation of Knowing to Thinking. In Griffiths A P (ed.) *Knowledge and Belief,* pp. 16–27. Oxford: Oxford University Press. Originally published in *Statement and Inference* by J Cook Wilson. Vol I, Part I, Section II, pp. 34–47. Oxford: Clarendon Press.

Witten I H, Frank E, Hall M A, and Pal C J (2017) *Data Mining: Practical Machine Learning Tools and Techniques.* 4th edition. Cambridge: Morgan Kaufmann.

Wittgenstein L (1969) *The Blue and Brown Books: Preliminary Studies for 'Philosophical Investigations'.* Oxford: Basil Blackwell.

Young J (2007) Editorial: Statistical errors in medical research – a chronic disease? *Swiss Medical Weekly.* 137(03–04), 41–43.

Zeitland I M (1997) *Ideology and The Development of Sociological Theory,* 6th edition. New Jersey: Prentice Hall.

Zellner B, Boerst C J, and Tabb W (2007) Statistics used in current nursing research. *Journal of Nursing Education.* 46(2), 55–59.

Ziliak S (2017) P values and the search for significance: Little P value, what are you trying to say of significance? Points of significance. *Nature Methods.* 14(1), 3–4.

INDEX

Note: Page numbers followed by 'n' refer to notes

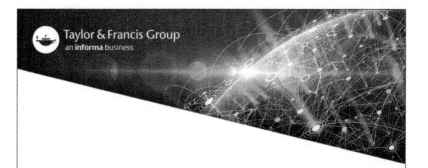